I0505320

ALTERNATIVE MEDICINE

DR. NASSER AFIFY

2019

TABLE OF CONTENTS

Introduction

Alternative medicine is the term for medical products and practices that are not part of standard care. Standard care is what medical doctors, doctors of osteopathy, and allied health professionals, such as nurses and physical therapists, practice. Alternative medicine is used in place of standard medical care. An example is treating heart disease with chelation therapy (which seeks to remove excess metals from the blood) instead of using a standard approach. Examples of alternative practices include homeopathy, traditional medicine, chiropractic, and acupuncture. Complementary medicine is different from alternative medicine. Whereas complementary medicine is used together with conventional medicine, alternative medicine is used in place of conventional medicine. See also complementary medicine, conventional medicine.

Something big is happening in healthcare, and it's centered on a desire to have different options within healthcare that considers the whole person. This demand is being filled by alternative medicine and a growing base of practitioners who are dedicated to leading the holistic healthcare movement. For instance, in 2012, Americans spent over $30 billion on alternative medicine. An estimated 59 million Americans spent an average of $500 per person on complementary and alternative medicine (CAM). From yoga to nutritional supplements to acupuncture, consumers across the nation are seeking alternatives to pharmaceutical drugs and surgery. Individuals turn to alternative medicine for various reasons. Some agree with the philosophy of Traditional Chinese Medicine, and some would like to expand their treatment options, while others are simply frustrated by the failure of conventional medicine to cure their illnesses. Alternative medicine is a subject of growing discussion within the healthcare industry. Skeptics of alternative medicine often perceive a lack of scientific evidence supporting alternative treatment options compared with the studies backing drugs and surgeries offered by conventional medicine. This skepticism has drawn researchers to conduct studies on treatments such as acupuncture, massage therapy, meditation, and yoga. Those occupying a middle ground conclude that though some treatments have sufficient evidence supporting their healing potential, patients should be wary of blindly accepting all alternative treatment options.

Healthcare education has seen an increase in the number of medical colleges offering programs and courses in alternative medicine. According to a report published by the National Center for Biotechnology Information (NCBI), 50.8 percent of 130 U.S. medical school websites that were systematically analyzed for course listings and content offered at least one CAM course or clerkship. The American Association of Naturopathic Medical Colleges (AANMC) has accredited seven naturopathic programs across eight North American campuses. The Council of Colleges of Acupuncture and Oriental Medicine have accredited 57 acupuncture schools, including the Pacific College of Oriental Medicine.

Consumer interest in preventive care and alternative treatment options has driven growth in the market for supplements and self-care. According to the National Center for Health Statistics, spending on natural product supplements was $12.8 billion in 2012, and spending on self-care approached $2.7 billion. According to McKinsey research, the U.S. vitamins, minerals, and nutritional and herbal supplements (VHMS) market was roughly 28 percent of the global market in 2013, which was valued at $82 billion. Expected growth in the VHMS market is between 5 and 6 percent per year, both in the U.S. and globally. This interest in disease prevention has already significantly increased consumer demand for the services of the nutritionists and dietitians industry and will likely continue to do so at a fast clip.

Complementary and alternative medicine, sometimes referred to as CAM, is an umbrella term for a vast array of treatments that fall outside conventional Western approaches. Some have been well-studied and proven to be effective; others have not.Although labels like "alternative medicine," "naturopathic medicine" and "integrative medicine" are often casually used (and misused), each term refers to something specific and different.

According to the National Center for Complementary and Integrative Health, actual alternative medicine is very rare. The organization defines alternative medicine as any non-conventional interventions that are used instead of conventional treatments, not in conjunction with them. Interventions like yoga, acupuncture, herbal remedies and massage therapy may be alternative treatments, but are considered alternative medicine only when they're used in place of conventional treatments, explained National Center for Complementary and Integrative Health Deputy Director David Shortleaf.

1. Types and methods of alternative medicine

-Acupressure

Acupressure is "a massage technique using the fingers and palms with a certain degree of force to stimulate acupoints and meridian lines on the surface of the skin. The purposes of acupressure are to regulate and balance the body energy or Qi and further to maintain health, prevent illness or enhance health" (Cho and Tsay, 2004). Acupressure is similar to acupuncture in that it selects particular points on the body.

Pressing on certain points is thought to "alter the internal flow of energy" (Collins and Thomas, 2004). It is an easy and convenient practice in that acupressure can be carried out by a practitioner or the patient himself. This method is commonly used to treat nausea and vomiting in chemotherapy patients. It is also utilized in the promotion of healthy blood flow. And in a small scale trial involving sixty-two patients, acupressure was effective in the treatment.

Acupuncture involves stimulating particular points on the body, and penetrating the skin with needles (Barnes, 2008). Supporting the use of acupuncture, "In 1997, after reviewing the available research, the NIH issued a consensus statement that acupuncture is effective for postoperative dental pain and for nausea and vomiting caused by anesthesia, chemotherapy, or pregnancy" (Collins and Thomas, 2004). Acupuncture is suggested to alleviate various pains or issues. Some of these include lower back pain, headaches, migraines, menstrual cramps, carpal tunnel syndrome, muscle pain, fibromyalgia, dental pain, and tendinitis (Collins and Thomas).

Trials from certified acupuncturists suggest that this treatment method may be effective in reducing pain or inflammation in osteoarthritis in the knee (Itoh, 2008). Various studies have also proposed that acupuncture may aid in treating asthma, as well as nausea and vomiting from chemotherapy. Trials are continually being conducted by various research groups, including the National Center for Complementary and Alternative Medicine, researching the efficacy of acupuncture in hypertension, heart failure, osteoarthritis, and opioid additions (Collins and Thomas).

-Aromatherapy

Aromatherapy involves the use of essential oils in stimulating olfactory receptors to elicit a response. Some common essential oils include chamomile, clary sage, lavender, and major am, Melissa, geranium, and rose (Han et al., 2006). Aromatherapy utilizes diffusers, baths, massages, and compresses. Because it is all natural elements and does not involve anything entering the body, aromatherapy is considered safe. Aromatherapy is asserted to stimulate circulation, stimulate the adrenocortical region, alleviate pain, reduce bleeding, and function as a sedative. In a small scale study involving the treatment of severe menstrual cramps, aromatherapy held promising results. In addition, most users hold claim to the effectiveness of this CAM method. However, "the therapeutic effects of aromatherapy are not well supported by clinical studies" (Han et al.).

-Ayurveda

Less known in western society, ayurveda is a traditional system of medicine from India. This treatment utilizes herbs as well as prepared herbal drugs. The goals are treatment, prevention, and improving the quality of life of the patient (Vayalil, 2002). According to ancient documentation, ayurveda is claimed to "arrests aging, enhance intelligence, memory, strength, youth, luster, sweetness of voice, and vigor" (Vayalil). Acting as antioxidants and enhancing the immune system, Ayurveda treatments are proposed to "nourish blood, lymph, flesh, adipose tissue, and semen and thus prevent degenerative changes and illness" (Vayalil). Despite the promising claims, little research or evidence is available to support the efficacy of this method.

-Biofeedback

Biofeedback involves improving an individual's overall health by training him to "consciously regulate bodily functions, such as breathing, heart rate, and blood pressure" (Barnes, 2008). It may use electomyographical or thermal methods. Biofeedback works to "increase awareness" in an individual of a particular "physiological process" (Thornton, 2002). An individual may learn what is acceptable by receiving a reward when a desired action or outcome is performed. Or a person may receive a punishment or "inhibition signal" when an adverse behavior or reaction occurs (Thornton). Biofeedback is oftentimes utilized for the safety of patients, or by patients who do not desire to take drugs, such as children (Termine, 2011). Common uses for this treatment include reduction of headaches and for the "clinical symptoms of puborectalis dyssynergia" (Zhu, 2011).

-Chelation

The goal of chelation is to tightly bind to and eliminate excess iron or toxic concentrations of other metals or minerals from the body. This method is frequently utilized by thalassemia patients, whose bodies do not produce enough normal red blood cells to eliminate these harmful elements (Delea, 2007). In one trial, chelation was employed in an attempt to eliminate lead in the blood of affected children. The experiment, however, demonstrated that chelation alone was not sufficient to lower the concentration of lead in children's blood to an acceptable level (Kassa, 2000). Though only limited trials have been conducted, chelation therapy has been approved for controlled use by the United States Food and Drug Administration (Delea).

-Chiropractic

Chiropractic treatment involves the manipulation of the spine and joints (Barnes, 2008). Various methods are used in chiropractic manipulation. However, like many other CAM methods, there is little specific evidence or data to support claims of efficacy (Gatterman, 2001). A study published in 2006 suggested that chiropractic care may be effective in "influencing the complex process of proprioceptive sensibility and pain of cervical origin" (Palmgren, 2006).

-Diet

Diet is one of the most commonly used forms of complementary and alternative medicine. Proper diet may be vital in preventing obesity, diabetes, or heart disease.

Diet involves an individualized treatment, because each person responds to diets differently. As opposed to using diet as a treatment, this method is most commonly a preventative treatment. As a result, in order for this method to be effective, focus would be required to shift to prevention. Most likely, this method would gain prevalence due to economic factors as opposed to experimental data (Williams, 2003).

-Dietary Supplement

Creative, protein powders, and other performance enhancements are commonly used as dietary supplements. Dietary supplements are "a product (other than tobacco) intended to supplement the diet that bears or contains one or more of the following ingredients: a vitamin, mineral, herb or other botanical, an amino acid, a dietary substance for use by humans to supplement the diet by increasing total daily intake, or a concentrate, metabolite, constituent, extract or combination of these ingredients" (Housman, 2011). Previously controlled by the Food and Drug Administration, dietary supplements are now available over the counter. Despite their prevalent use, "consumption of unregulated dietary supplements has been associated with adverse effects (i.e., heavy metal poisoning, heart-related health issues, and hyperthermia)" (Housman).

-Energy Healing

Beginning with research involving electricity and wound healing in the 1940s, energy healing gained popularity in the 1950s. Pulse electromagnetic energy gives "the tissues an energy boost in the form of an electromagnetic field without the tissues being required to tolerate a thermal load" (McGaughey, 2009).

Some theories propose that energy healing functions by assisting with phagocytic and enzyme activity within cell membranes, as well as possibly influencing ion flow and cell membrane potential. In addition, "The physiological effects are thought to include: an increase in the number of white cells and fibroblasts in a wound, improved rate of edema dispersion and reabsorption of hematomas, reduction of inflammation, enhanced deposition and organization of collagen and fibrin, stimulation of ontogenesis and enhanced blood flow" (McGaughey). Little research involving energy healing has been conducted, and there is even less convincing evidence for its efficacy.

-Folk Remedies

Are generally passed down culturally or generationally, and involve herbs, food products, or household items. Common remedies for diseases or issues include drugs (acetaminophen, ibuprofen, and benzocaine), cool baths, potatoes or onions in socks, sienna extract, chamomile, steam, covering the head, massages, whiskey for teething, ice cubes, vanilla, or clove.

Additionally, laxatives (cod liver oil, castor oil, senna) and diuretics (herbal tea) are common. In the past, "folk remedy use has been associated with a lack of access to health care because of a shortage of physicians, language or cultural barriers, socioeconomic status, or mistrust of physicians" (Smitherman, 2005).

Now, folk remedies are utilized because of their perceived effectiveness or cultural acceptance. Because physicians or medical professionals are often not consulted before folk remedy regiments are instituted, potential harm may occur. For example, remedies involving isopropyl alcohol may cause poisoning if absorbed by the skin or inhaled (Smitherman).

-Herbal Therapy

Herbal therapies are generally accepted as safe. The main purpose is for an individual's general wellness or treatment of a particular illness. Common herbal therapies include garlic, chamomile, Echinacea, milk thistle, ginseng, aloe vera, dandelion root, and cats claw (Johnson, 2000). Like many other CAM methods, few trials have been conducted evaluating the efficacy of herbal therapy. Homeopathy Homeopathic theory is based on the principle that substances that cause certain symptoms in high doses can cure the same symptoms in low doses. Commonly used substances include Arsenicum album, Calcarea carbonica, Chamomilla, Podophyllum, and sulphur (Jacobs, 2006). Definite evidence has yet to be proven, because, in general, the evidence for the effectiveness of homeopathic combination remedies has been inconclusive.

Some studies have shown that combination remedies are effective in treating rheumatoid arthritis, sea sickness, and vertigo, whereas others have shown them to be ineffective in the treatment of plantar warts and postoperative ileus" (Jacobs). Because various studies of homeopathy did not publish negative data, bias involving the effectiveness of this treatment is brought into question (Linde, 1998).

Humor though not typically perceived as a treatment, humor can often be an effective means of mood change or coping mechanisms. It can make situations appear more positive, so as to avoid death, depression, or suicide. According to a study from 2007, "Therapeutic humor results in decreased anxiety and the pleasure of being able to laugh at what is feared, but telling funny jokes is not the essence of therapeutic humor" (Richman, 2007).

Therapeutic humor in medicine does not involve laughing at situations of death, depression, anxiety, or panic. Instead, it makes light of the situation and replaces the unpleasant emotions that were formerly looming. The goal is to "reduce stress and affirm life" (Richman).

- Hypnosis

Hypnosis attempts to alter an individual's state of consciousness, relying on the principle of suggestion. It is often used to treat anxiety disorder or post-traumatic stress disorders. Hypnosis is centered on a person's perception and redirecting his attention away from a particular issue. But despite any evidence in favor of hypnosis, it is often argued that "suggestive effects in medicine are discounted as placebo effects" (Mende, 2009).

Essentially, this would make this entire method invalid. Imagery is described as "a highly focused form of concentration that creates an alteration of sensations, awareness, and perceptions with the same biopsychosocial, integrative properties that allow people to process sensory information" (Wynd, 2005). Imagery is most commonly used in relation to surgery, cancer chemotherapy, reducing burn pain, headache, rheumatoid arthritis, chronic pain, rape, assault, and motivation for exercise. This method often times appears successful.

-Iridology

Iridology involves studying part of the eye in order to diagnose diseases or issues found throughout the body. Iridologists believe that particular points on the iris surface correspond with certain organs in the body. They consider the color, pigment, and other features in order to diagnose a patient. Additionally, they claim that if an organ has been affected, a mark or scar will be visible on the iris. According to some experts, they could clearly view carcinomas of the breast, ovary, uterus, prostate, and colorectal when observing the iris (Munstedt, 2005).

However, in a study conducted in 2005 involving iridology and cancer, "the results clearly show that iridology did not identify the cancer patients at an acceptable statistical level. Patients with two different malignancies were also not identified correctly. For the various benign diseases, iridology was of no help. Additional statistical cross correlation analyses confirmed these findings. In addition, analysis of other benign diseases, which was not part of our initial study design, and the correlation to iridologic findings, failed to show that

iridology was useful in detecting these disorders"
(Mundstedt).

2. Use of Complementary and Alternative Medicine in Europe

Complementary and alternative medicine (CAM) has become more popular and accepted in Europe which reflects trends observed in other western countries. Although this development has been acknowledged in European health policies, the knowledge base for informed policy actions is limited, and further evidence on the prevalence and determinants of CAM use in Europe is required. Many existing CAM studies suffer from methodological shortcomings, including inadequate operational definitions, recall bias related to long timeframes of the survey measures and insufficient coverage of European countries.

Moreover, most studies have reported only unadjusted associations, which neglect potential confounding variables. Consequently, cross-country comparisons of CAM utilization are difficult, and prevalence estimates vary greatly, even in the case of single countries. Moreover, although there is a considerable body of CAM research in some countries, such as the UK and Germany, there is a lack of evidence of CAM use in many others, especially Eastern European countries.

According to a review by Yeardley et al., the most frequently used CAM modalities in Europe are herbal medicine, homeopathy, chiropractic, acupuncture and reflexology. Massage was also found to be a widely used CAM treatment. Typically, CAM is used to complement biomedical care. With regard to sociodemographics, CAM users are more likely to be female, better educated and middle-aged. In terms of health determinants, Yeardley et al. found that musculoskeletal problems were the most common condition treated with CAM. Reviewing the global CAM literature, Fras et al. reported that back problems, depression, insomnia, severe headaches or migraines and stomach or intestinal illnesses were the most typical conditions associated with CAM.

Some previous studies investigated CAM use for specific health problems or illnesses, such as multiple sclerosis and cancer. Menniti-Ippolito et al. found that, in Italy, acupuncture and manipulative therapies were primarily used for alleviating pain, whereas herbal medicine was more often employed to improve quality of life. In contrast, the use of homeopathy was not associated with any specific health problems.

In addition to its use in medical conditions, some typical motivations for CAM use are relaxation, improvements in subjective wellbeing, preventive care, a preference for natural care instead of biomedical medicine, a desire for more personalized and holistic care, dissatisfaction with biomedicine and dissatisfaction with the doctor-patient relationship. The heterogeneity of an individual's social network, resulting in exposure to a wide range of information and values, was also found to increase the probability of using CAM.

In practical terms, this study is of help to both medical professionals and CAM providers, as it provides information on the medical conditions for which CAM is most often used. A comprehensive medical history is paramount to quality care, but patients do not always inform healthcare professionals about CAM use, which can lead to harmful double treatment or medication.

The study also offers information for CAM providers on the medical backgrounds of their clients. They can utilize this information to ensure safe care and assess the need for biomedical care. CAM is an economic and societal issue related to money spent on treatments, the relationship between CAM and public healthcare and inequalities in health service use.

This study utilized data from the European Social Survey, Round 7 (edition 2.0, 2014), which is a biennial cross-sectional survey project using face-to-face interviews. In the case of the Czech Republic, data on cancer were lacking, and data on other medical conditions in Estonia were missing. Consequently, these countries were excluded from the respective analyses. The data included post-stratification weights to account for the sampling design and address the implications of non-response.

Using dichotomous survey items, the respondents were asked about their use of different healthcare modalities during the last 12 months. The CAM items were acupuncture, acupressure, Chinese medicine, chiropractic, osteopathy, homeopathy, herbal treatment, hypnotherapy, massage therapy, reflexology and spiritual healing. The survey also recorded data on the respondents' use of physiotherapy and consultation with a general practitioner or medical specialist.

Our CAM classification draws on the widely accepted approach of the National Institutes of Health (NIH) and National Center for Complementary and Alternative Medicine (NCCAM) with slight modifications following Fulder. We distinguished four categories of CAM treatments. First, we used the category of traditional Asian medical systems (TAMS), which can be described as 'complete system[s] of theory and practice', having evolved independently from biomedical medicine. In the present study, this category included traditional Chinese medicine, acupuncture and acupressure. Second, drawing on Fulder, we constructed an alternative medicinal systems (AMS) category, which refers to the intake of substances thought to have healing potential. These systems included homeopathy and herbal treatment. The third category was manual body-based therapies, which involve body movements and focus on the structures and systems of the body.

This category comprised massage therapy, chiropractic, osteopathy and reflexology. The final category was mind-body therapies, which emphasize the role of thought and emotion in healing. This category included hypnotherapy and spiritual healing. We created a dichotomous variable for each CAM category (i.e. used a treatment in a given category during the last 12 months vs not). Some other CAM therapies, such as energy therapies and nature cure therapies were not included in the survey data.

Health problems during the last 12 months were indicated with dichotomous items. The items included heart or circulatory problems, high blood pressure, breathing problems, allergies, back or neck pain, upper extremity pain, lower extremity pain, stomach or digestive system problems, skin conditions, severe headaches and diabetes. The item on cancer covered current disease and previous occurrences, and here they were combined in one category. Depression was measured using an eight-item version of the CES-D scale. The items were feelings of depression, everything is an effort, loneliness, happiness, sadness, enjoyment in life, restless sleep and could not get 'going' during the past week. The items were marked on a four-point scale, ranging from 'none' or 'almost none of the time' to 'all' or 'almost all the time'. The sum was dichotomized between 8 and 9, corresponding to the cutoff point used commonly in longer scales.

Finally, standard sociodemographic control variables included gender, age (categorized), education (International Standard Classification of Education), household's total net income (docile) and country, with Hungary selected as the reference due to its low level of CAM use.

Percentages and their confidence intervals as well as logistic regression models were estimated using the Complex Samples module of SPSS 22. In the text, 5% was used as the level of statistical significance. We controlled for the standard sociodemographic factors and country. Also, comorbidity was controlled for by including all the health variables in the models. To retain analytic power, the missing values of the household variable (n=8296) were included in the logistic regression models as a separate category. The analyses were conducted using a survey weight variable that combines the post-stratification and country weights, except in those analyses that included country as an analytical variable. In these cases the country was already controlled for and the post-stratification weights were sufficient. The use of mind-body therapies was a relatively rare outcome, but comparing the maximum likelihood results with those from penalized estimation, run in R, suggests that the number of events was sufficient and, thus, the ordinary estimates could be relied on.

The most frequently used CAM treatment was massage therapy, used by 11.9% of the population, followed by homeopathy (5.7%), osteopathy (5.2%), herbal treatments (4.6%), acupuncture (3.6%), chiropractic (2.3%), reflexology (1.7%) and spiritual healing (1.3%). Other modalities (Chinese medicine, acupressure and hypnotherapy) were used by around by 1% or less.

In the case of manual therapies, as expected, back or neck pain as well as pain in the upper and lower extremity was associated with this type of care. The presence of allergies, heart and circulatory problems and stomach and digestive system problems were also significant predictors of the use of manual therapies. Finally, mind-body therapies were commonly used by those with stomach or digestive system problems and those with cancer. It is noteworthy that mind-body care was the only CAM modality associated with depression. The presence of severe headaches, allergies, back or neck pain and upper extremity pain was also associated with the use of mind-body therapies.

Back and neck pain, stomach and digestive system problems, upper extremity pain and allergies were strong predictors of CAM use in all categories. High blood pressure had no independent predictive power in any of the models. With regard to income, those with a lower income were more likely to be users of mind-body therapies. In contrast, those with a higher income were more inclined to be users of the other three CAM modalities.

In terms of country-level differences, the highest ORs for the use of TAMS were found in Denmark, Switzerland and Israel, followed by Austria, Norway and Sweden. The highest OR for the use of AMS was found in Lithuania, while manual therapies were most commonly used in Finland, Austria, Switzerland, Germany and Denmark. Moreover, Denmark, Ireland, Slovenia and Lithuania had the highest ORs for using mind-body therapies. France, Spain and Germany presented a common pattern, with relatively similar use of the different modalities. Poland and Hungary had low ORs for use of the different CAM modalities.

The more prevalent CAM use in pain- and allergy-related conditions may reflect their ambiguous and uncertain character, which may leave patients without a clear understanding of causes and remedies. In these cases, CAM use may function as a coping strategy against this kind of uncertainty. In contrast with the findings of a previous study, people with depression were not the most active CAM users. This may be because finding information and making an informed decision on treatment can be difficult due to hampered agency.

In the present study, the use of CAM varied greatly by country. The variation can be partly explained by regulations governing the use of CAM and the inclusion of CAM in biomedical practice and health insurance. For example, in Germany and Switzerland, some forms of CAM are covered by insurance. In Austria, where CAM use is high, general practitioners receive training in CAM methods. Some country-level differences may also be cultural.

For example, in large multicultural countries, such as France and Germany, the use of different CAM modalities is widespread, whereas this is not the case in the more homogeneous Nordic countries. Furthermore, the diffusion of ideas in German-speaking countries may partly explain the higher usage of AMS, including homeopathy, which originated in Germany.

In relation to previous CAM studies, the key strengths of this study stem from the comparable findings on the surveyed European countries, its focus on different CAM modalities and the association of these modalities with different health problems, in addition to the multiple regression approach used to control for confounding variation. On the other hand, it is well known that cross-sectional data do not allow for optimal estimation of causal impacts. In addition, the study did not include all known CAM treatment modalities, which may lead to underestimation of CAM usage rates. Furthermore, data were not available on the frequency of CAM use. Thus, it was not possible to distinguish the single use of CAM therapy versus more frequent usage. Finally, country-level differences may exist in what is considered complementary or alternative care.

In conclusion, our study demonstrated that CAM was commonly used for health-related problems in Europe. Hence, CAM should not be viewed as a form of relaxation or preventive care used only by those in good health. CAM was not used as a sole alternative to biomedical care. Instead, it was typically used in a complementary manner. The patterns of help-seeking behavior differed according to the health-related problem.

For example, those suffering from pain conditions turned to a wide range of CAM treatment modalities. On the other hand, AMS especially attracts help-seekers with various medical conditions, which should be taken into account by the providers of these treatments in order to provide safe care. In addition, individuals in a higher socioeconomic position were more likely to turn to a wider range of CAM options than individuals in a lower socioeconomic position. Therefore, those with a higher socioeconomic status were more likely than those with a lower socioeconomic status to find a satisfactory combination of biomedical and complementary therapies. This finding points towards a possible socioeconomic inequality in health service use.

3. The use of alternative medicine in Africa

Traditional medicine is the sum total of knowledge, skills, and practices based on the theories, beliefs, and experiences indigenous to different cultures that are used to maintain health, as well as to prevent, diagnose, improve, or treat physical and mental illnesses. Traditional medicine that has been adopted by other populations (outside its indigenous culture) is often termed complementary or alternative medicine (CAM).

The World Health Organization (WHO) reported that 80% of the emerging world's population relies on traditional medicine for therapy. During the past decades, the developed world has also witnessed an ascending trend in the utilization of CAM, particularly herbal remedies. Herbal medicines include herbs, herbal materials, herbal preparations, and finished herbal products that contain parts of plants or other plant materials as active ingredients. While 90% of the population in Ethiopia use herbal remedies for their primary healthcare, surveys carried out in developed countries like Germany and Canada tend to show that at least 70% of their population have tried CAM at least once. It is likely that the profound knowledge of herbal remedies in traditional cultures, developed through trial and error over many centuries, along with the most important cures was carefully passed on verbally from one generation to another. Indeed, modern allopathic medicine has its roots in this ancient medicine, and it is likely that many important new remedies will be developed and commercialized in the future from the African biodiversity, as it has been till now, by following the leads provided by traditional knowledge and experiences.

The extensive use of traditional medicine in Africa, composed mainly of medicinal plants, has been argued to be linked to cultural and economic reasons. This is why the WHO encourages African member states to promote and integrate traditional medical practices in their health system. Plants typically contain mixtures of different phytochemicals, also known as secondary metabolites that may act individually, additively, or in synergy to improve health. Indeed, medicinal plants, unlike pharmacological drugs, commonly have several chemicals working together catalytically and synergistically to produce a combined effect that surpasses the total activity of the individual constituents. The combined actions of these substances tend to increase the activity of the main medicinal constituent by speeding up or slowing down its assimilation in the body. Secondary metabolites from plant's origins might increase the stability of the active compound or phytochemicals, minimize the rate of undesired adverse side effects, and have an additive, potentiating, or antagonistic effect. It has been postulated that the enormous diversity of chemical structures found in these plants is not waste products, but specialized secondary metabolites involved in the relationship of the organism with the environment, for example, attractants of pollinators, signal products, defensive substances against predators and parasites, or in resistance against pests and diseases. A single plant may, for example, contain bitter substances that stimulate digestion and possess anti-inflammatory compounds that reduce swellings and pain, phenolic compounds that can act as an antioxidant and venotonics, antibacterial and antifungal tannins that act as natural antibiotics, diuretic substances that enhance the elimination of waste products and toxins, and alkaloids that enhance mood and give a sense of well-being.

Although some may view the isolation of phytochemicals and their use as single chemical entities as a better alternative and which have resulted in the replacement of plant extracts' use, nowadays, a view that there may be some advantages of the medical use of crude and/or standardized extracts as opposed to isolated single compound is gaining much momentum in the scientific community.

-African Traditional Medicine

African traditional medicine is the oldest, and perhaps the most assorted, of all therapeutic systems. Africa is considered to be the cradle of mankind with a rich biological and cultural diversity marked by regional differences in healing practices. African traditional medicine in its varied forms is holistic involving both the body and the mind. The traditional healer typically diagnoses and treats the psychological basis of an illness before prescribing medicines, particularly medicinal plants to treat the symptoms. The sustained interest in traditional medicine in the African healthcare system can be justified by two major reasons. The first one is inadequate access to allopathic medicines and western forms of treatments, whereby the majority of people in Africa cannot afford access to modern medical care either because it is too costly or because there are no medical service providers. Second, there is a lack of effective modern medical treatment for some ailments such as malaria and/or which, although global in distribution, disproportionately affects Africa more than other areas in the world.

The most common traditional medicine in common practice across the African continent is the use of medicinal plants. In many parts of Africa, medicinal plants are the most easily accessible health resource available to the community. In addition, they are most often the preferred option for the patients. For most of these people, traditional healers offer information, counseling, and treatment to patients and their families in a personal manner as well as having an understanding of their patient's environment. Indeed, Africa is blessed with enormous biodiversity resources and it is estimated to contain between 40 and 45,000 species of plant with a potential for development and out of which 5,000 species are used medicinally. This is not surprising since Africa is located within the tropical and subtropical climate and it is a known fact that plants accumulate important secondary metabolites through evolution as a natural means of surviving in a hostile environment. Because of her tropical conditions, Africa has an unfair share of strong ultraviolet rays of the tropical sunlight and numerous pathogenic microbes, including several species of bacteria, fungi, and viruses, suggesting that African plants could accumulate chemo preventive substances more than plants from the northern hemisphere. Interestingly, Abegaz et al. have observed that of all species of Dorstenia (Moraceae) analyzed, only the African species, Dorstenia mania Hook's, a perennial herb growing in the tropical rain forest of Central Africa contained more biological activity than related species.

Nonetheless, the documentation of medicinal uses of African plants and traditional systems is becoming a pressing need because of the rapid loss of the natural habitats of some of these plants due to anthropogenic activities and also due to an erosion of valuable traditional knowledge. It has been reported that Africa has some 216 million hectares of forest, but the African continent is also notorious to have one of the highest rates of deforestation in the world, with a calculated loss through deforestation of 1% per annum. Interestingly, the continent also has the highest rate of endemism, with the Republic of Madagascar topping the list by 82%, and it is worth to emphasize that Africa already contributes nearly 25% of the world trade in biodiversity. Nonetheless, the paradox is that in spite of this huge potential and diversity, the African continent has only few drugs commercialized globally.

The scientific literature has witnessed a growing number of publications geared towards evaluating the efficacy of medicinal plants from Africa which are believed to have an important contribution in the maintenance of health and in the introduction of new treatments. Nonetheless, there is still a dearth of updated comprehensive compilation of promising medicinal plants from the African continent.

The main aim of the present review is to highlight the importance and potential of medicinal plants from the African biodiversity which have short- as well as long-term potential to be developed as future phytopharmaceuticals to treat and/or manage panoply of infectious and chronic conditions. The review might also provide a starting point for future studies aimed at isolation, purification, and characterization of bioactive compounds present in these plants as well as exploring the potential niche market of these plants. In this endeavor, major scientific databases such as EBSCOhost, PubMed Central, Scopus (Elsevier), and Emerald amongst others have been probed to investigate trends in the rapidly increasing number of scientific publications on African traditional medicinal plants. Ten medicinal plants (Acacia senegal, Aloe ferox, Artemisia herba-alba, Aspalathus linearis, Centella asiatica, Catharanthus roseus, Cyclopia genistoides, Harpagophytum procumbens, Momordica charantia, and Pelargonium sidoides) of special interest were chosen for more detailed reviews based on the following criteria: medicinal plants that form part of African herbal pharmacopeia with commercial importance and those plants from which modern phytopharmaceuticals have been derived.

Acacia Senegal, also known as gum Arabic, is native to semi desert and drier regions of sub-Saharan Africa, but widespread from Southern to Northern Africa. It is used as a medicinal plant in parts of Northern Nigeria, West Africa, North Africa, and other parts of the world. The use of gum Arabic (or gum acacia), which is derived from an exudate from the bark, dates from the first Egyptian Dynasty (3400 B.C.). It was used in the production of ink, which was made from a mixture of carbon, gum, and water. Inscriptions from the 18th Dynasty refer to this gum as "komi" or "komme." Gum Arabic has been used for at least 4,000 years by local people for the preparation of food, in human and veterinary medicine, in crafts, and as a cosmetic. The gum of A. Senegal has been used medicinally for centuries, and various parts of the plant are used to treat infections such as bleeding, bronchitis, diarrhea, gonorrhea, leprosy, typhoid fever, and upper respiratory tract infections. African herbalists use gum acacia to bind pills and to stabilize emulsions. It is also used in aromatherapy for applying essential oils.

Currently, A. Senegal is an important naturally occurring oil-in-water emulsifier, which is in regular use in the food and pharmaceutical industries. Medicinally, gum Arabic is used extensively in pharmaceutical preparations and is a food additive approved as toxicologically safe by the Codex Aliment Arius. It has been used as demulcent, skin protective agent, and pharmaceutical aids such as emulsifier and stabilizer of suspensions and additives for solid formulations. It is sometimes used to treat bacterial and fungal infections of the skin and mouth. It has been reported to soothe the mucous membranes of the intestines and to treat inflamed skin.

The demulcent, emollient gum is used internally against inflammation of intestinal mucosa and externally to cover inflamed surfaces, as burns, sore nipples, and nodular leprosy. Additionally, it has also been documented to be used as antitussive, expectorant, astringent, catarrh and against colds, coughs, diarrhea, dysentery, gonorrhea, hemorrhage, sore throat, typhoid, and for urinary tract ailments. The gum of A. Senegal has been pharmaceutically used mainly in the manufacture of emulsions and in making pills and troches (as an excipient), as demulcent for inflammations of the throat or stomach and as masking agent for acrid tasting substances such as capsicum and also as a film-forming agent in peel-off masks. Gum Arabic is also used widely as an ingredient in foods like candies and soft drinks as the gum has the properties of glue that is safe to eat. Gum acacia is widely used in organic products as natural alternative to chemical binders and is used in commercial emulsification for the production of beverages and flavor concentrates.

Recently, it has been reported that A. Senegal bark extracts were evaluated in vitro for their antimicrobial potential against human pathogenic isolates (Escherichia coli, Staphylococcus aurous, Streptococcus pneumoniae, Klebsiella pneumoniae, Shigella dysenteriae, Salmonella typhi, Streptococcus pyogenes, Pseudomonas aeruginosa, and Proteus vulgaris). The extract was found to exhibit significant antibacterial activity which was suggested to be due to the presence of tannins and saponins in the plant. It was also reported that the plant extract may not be toxic to man following in vitro cytotoxicity evaluation.

Aloe ferox is native to South Africa and Lesotho and is considered to be the most common Aloe species in South Africa. A. ferox has been used since time immemorial and has a well-documented history of use as an alternative medicine and is one of the few plants depicted in San rock paintings. The bitter latex, known as Cape aloe, is used as laxative medicine in Africa and Europe and is considered to have bitter tonic, antioxidant, anti-inflammatory, antimicrobial, and anticancer properties.

The use of A. ferox as a multipurpose traditional medicine has been translated into several commercial applications and it is a highly valued plant in the pharmaceutical, natural health, food, and cosmetic industries. A. ferox is considered South Africa's main wild harvested commercially traded species. The finished product obtained from aloe tapping, aloe bitters, has remained a key South African export product since 1761 when it was first exported to Europe. The aloe tapping industry is the livelihood of many rural communities and formalization of the industry in the form of establishment of cooperatives and trade agreements. It has been suggested that its trade may have an extensive poverty alleviation effect in Africa.

A. ferox has many traditional and documented medicinal uses. It is most popularly used for its laxative effect and as a topical application to the skin, eyes, and mucous membranes. Scientific studies conducted have verified many of the traditional uses. More recently, the cosmetic industry has shown interest in A. ferox gel. It has been reported that A. ferox gel contains at least 130 medicinal agents with anti-inflammatory, analgesic, calming, antiseptic, germicidal, antiviral, antiparasitic, antitumour, and anticancer effects encompassing all of the traditional uses and scientific studies done on A. ferox and its constituents.

A wide variety of phenolic compounds (chromones, anthraquinones, anthrone, anthrone-C-glycosides, and other phenolic compounds) are present within A. ferox and these compounds have been well documented to possess biological activity. The gel polysaccharides are known to be of the arabinogalactan and rhamnogalacturonan types. The leaf gel composition still remains unknown and it's claimed biological activities still remain to be investigated. The active ingredient (purgative principle) is a chemical compound known as Aloin (also called Barbaloin).

The gel has also been found to be rich in antioxidant polyphenols, indoles, and alkaloids. Tests carried out have shown that the nonflavonoid polyphenols contribute to the majority of the total polyphenol content. With this phytochemical profile, A. ferox leaf gel has been identified to be very promising in alleviating symptoms associated with/or prevention of common no communicable diseases such as cardiovascular diseases, cancer, neurodegeneration, and diabetes.

The leaves have been reported to contain two juices; the yellow bitter sap is used as laxative while the white aloe gel is used in health drinks and skin care products. This purgative drug is used for stomach complaints, mainly as a laxative to "purify" the stomach and also as a bitter tonic (amarum) in various digestives and stomachics (such as "Lewensessens" and "Swedish Bitters"). Usually, a small crystal of the drug (0.05–0.2 g) is taken orally as a laxative. Half the laxative dose is suggested for arthritis.

The fresh bitter sap is instilled directly against conjunctivitis and sinusitis. It is well known that bitter substances stimulate the flow of gastric juices and in so doing improve digestion. The fresh juice emanating from the cut leaf is also applied on burn wounds. A. ferox is claimed to detoxify the damaged surface area and exhibit analgesic and anesthetic properties while promoting new tissue formation (granulation) which fills the wound. It was demonstrated that A. ferox enriched with aloins can inhibit collagenase and metalloprotease activity, which can degrade collagen connective tissues.

The effect of A. ferox whole leaf juice on wound healing and skin repair was investigated in an animal model and its safety was evaluated. The results showed that the A. ferox whole leaf juice preparation accelerates wound closure and selectively inhibits microbial growth. No dermal toxicity or side effects were observed during the experimental period.

Artemisia herba-alba is commonly known as wormwood or desert wormwood (known in Arabic as shih, and as Armoise Blanche in French). It is a grayish strongly aromatic perennial dwarf shrub native to the Northern Africa, Arabian Peninsula, and Western Asia. A. herba-alba has been used in folk medicine by many cultures since ancient times. In Moroccan folk medicine, it is used to treat arterial hypertension and diabetes and in Tunisia, it is used to treat diabetes, bronchitis, diarrhea, hypertension, and neuralgias. Herbal tea from A. herba-alba has been used as analgesic, antibacterial, antispasmodic, and hemostatic agents in folk medicines. During an ethno pharmacological survey carried out among the Bedouins of the Negev desert, it was found that A. herba-alba was used to mitigate stomach disorders. This plant is also suggested to be important as a fodder for sheep and for livestock in the plateau regions of Algeria where it grows abundantly. It has also been reported that Acaridae from hogs and ground worms were killed by the oil of the Libyan A. herba-alba in a short time.

Oral administration of 0.39 g/kg body weight of the aqueous extract of the leaves or barks of A. herba-alba has been documented to produce a significant reduction in blood glucose level, while the aqueous extract of roots and metabolic extract of the aerial parts of the plant produce almost no reduction in blood glucose level. The extract of the aerial parts of the plant seems to have minimal adverse effect and high LD50 value.

Among A. herba-alba phytochemical constituents, essential oils have been extensively studied, with several chemotypes being recognized. The variability from the essential oils isolated from A. herba-alba collected in Algeria, Israel, Morocco, and Spain was revised by Dob and Benabdelkader, but, since then, many other studies have reinforced its high chemical polymorphism. Recently, fifty components were identified in A. herba-alba oils, oxygen-containing monoterpenes being dominant in all cases (72–80%). Camphor (17–33%), α-thujone (7–28%), and chrysanthenone (4–19%) were the major oil components. Despite the similarity in main components, three types of oils could be defined: (a) α-thujone: camphor (23–28: 17–28%), (b) camphor: chrysanthenone (33 : 12%), and (c) α-thujone : camphor : chrysanthenone (24 : 19 : 19%).

The antifungal activity of Artemisia herba-alba was found to be associated with two major volatile compounds isolated from the fresh leaves of the plant. Carvone and piperitone were isolated from Artemisia herba-alba. The antifungal activity of the purified compounds carbon and piperitone was estimated to be 5 µg/mL and 2 µg/mL against Penicillium citrinum and 7 µg/mL and 1.5 µg/mL against Mucor rouxii, respectively. In another study, the antifungal activity of the constituents and biological activities of Artemisia herba-alba essential oils of 25 Moroccan medicinal plants, including A. herba-alba, against Penicillium digitatum, Phytophthora citrophthora, Geotrichum citri-aurantii, and Botrytis cinerea have been reported.

Aspalathus linearis, an endemic South African fibs species, is cultivated to produce the well-known herbal tea, also commonly known as rooibos. Its caffeine-free and comparatively low tannin status, combined with its potential health-promoting properties, most notably antioxidant activity, has contributed to its popularity and consumer acceptance globally. The utilization of rooibos has also moved beyond a herbal tea to intermediate value-added products such as extracts for the beverage, food, nutraceuticals and cosmetic markets.

Rooibos is used traditionally throughout Africa in numerous ways. It has been used as a refreshment drink and as a healthy tea beverage. It was only after the discovery that an infusion of rooibos, when administered to her colicky baby, cured the chronic restlessness, vomiting, and stomach cramps that rooibos became well known as a "healthy" beverage, leading to a broader consumer base. Many babies since then have been nurtured with rooibos—either added to their milk or given as a weak brew.

Animal studies have suggested that it has potent antioxidant, immunomodulation, and chemo preventive effects. The plant is rich in minerals and low in tannins. Among the flavonoids present are the unique C-glucoside dihydrochalcones: aspalathin and nothofagin and with aspalathin being the most abundant. In vitro data has shown that the daily intake of the alkaline extracts of the red rooibos tea could suppress HIV infections in the extract, though clinical evaluation has yet to be conducted.

There is growing evidence that the flavonoids present in the plant contribute substantially to a reduction in cardiovascular disease and other ailments associated with ageing. Recent studies have shown that aspalathin has beneficial effects on glucose homeostasis in Type 2 diabetes through stimulating glucose uptake in muscle tissues and insulin secretion from pancreatic beta-cells. The unfermented rooibos has been found to have greater chemo protective effects than the fermented variety. Aspalathin has free-radical capturing properties and is absorbed through the small intestine as such.

The bronchodilator, antispasmodic, and blood pressure lowering effects of rooibos tea have been confirmed in vitro and in vivo. It has also been reported that the antispasmodic effect of the rooibos is mediated predominantly through potassium ionchannel activation. There is also increasing evidence of antimutagenic effects. Animal study suggested the prevention of age-related accumulation of lipid peroxidases in the brain.

Rooibos is becoming more popular in western countries particularly among health-conscious consumers, due to the absence of alkaloids and low tannin content. It is also reported to have a high level of antioxidants such as aspalathin and nothofagin. The ant oxidative effect has also been attributed to the presence of water-soluble polyphenols such as ruin and quercetin. Rooibos is purported to assist nervous tension, allergies, and digestive problems.

Rooibos extracts, usually combined with other ingredients, are available in pill form, but these products fall in the category of dietary supplements. Recent research has underscored the potential of aspalathin and selected rooibos extracts such as an aspalathin-enriched green rooibos extract as antidiabetic agents. A patent application for the use of aspalathin in this context was filed in Japan, while a placebo-controlled trial application was filed for the use of rooibos extract as an antidiabetic agent. It is claimed that rooibos extract and a hetero-dimer containing aspalathin, isolated from rooibos, could be used as a drug for the treatment of neurological and psychiatric disorders of the central nervous system. Other opportunities may lie with topical skin products.

Two studies concerning inhibition of COX-2 in mouse skin and inhibition of mouse skin tumor promotion tend to support the role of the topical application of rooibos extract. Nonetheless, more research would be needed to explore its potential in preventing skin cancer in humans.

Centella asiatica is a medicinal plant that has been used since prehistoric times. It has a pan-tropical distribution and is used in many healing cultures, including Ayurvedic medicine, Chinese traditional medicine, Kampo (Japanese traditional medicine), and African traditional medicine. To date, it continues to be used within the structure of folk medicine and is increasingly being located at the interface between traditional and modern scientifically oriented medicine. Traditionally, C. asiatica is used mainly for wound healing, burns, ulcers, leprosy, tuberculosis, lupus, skin diseases, eye diseases, fever, inflammation, asthma, hypertension, rheumatism, syphilis, epilepsy, diarrhea, and mental illness and is also eaten as a vegetable or used as a spice. In Mauritius, the application of C. asiatica in the treatment of leprosy was reported for the first time in 1852 while the clinical use of C. asiatica, as a therapeutic agent suitable for the treatment of leprous lesions, has been documented since 1887.

The active constituents are characterized by their clinical effects in the treatment of chronic venous disease, wound healing, and cognitive functions amongst others. C. asiatica contains a variety of pentacyclic triterpenoids that have been extensively studied. Asiaticoside and madecassoside are the two most important active compounds that are used in drug preparations.

Both are commercially used mainly as wound-healing agent, based on their anti-inflammatory effects. One of the main active constituents of C. asiatica is the ursane-type triterpene saponin, asiaticoside, which is responsible for wound healing properties and is known to stimulate type 1 collagen synthesis in fibroblast cells. Plants collected from various geographical regions and locations in India, Madagascar, Malaysia, Sri Lanka, Andaman Islands, and South Africa have yielded concentrations of asiaticoside ranging from 0.006 to 6.42% of dry weight. C. asiatica also contains several other triterpene saponins. Madecassoside always co-occurs with asiaticoside as a main compound and other saponins have been reported, such as asiaticosides A to G, centelloside, brahmoside, and many others. Madagascar plays a major role in C. asiatica trade. It is the first producer of C. asiatica products worldwide and due to a higher Asiaticoside content of dried leaves; Malagasy origin is appreciated by industry.

The ethyl acetate fraction of C. asiatica has been reported to increase the effect of the imp. Administrated antiepileptic drugs phenytoin, valproate, and gabapentin and was found to decrease the pentylenetetrazol- (PTZ-) kindled induced seizures in rats.This effect might be due to an increase in gamma-aminobutyric acid (GABA) levels caused by the extract as reported by Chatterjee et al.

The neuroprotective properties of the plant in monosodium glutamate treated rats were investigated by Ramanathan et al. The general behavior, locomotor activity, and the CA1 region of the hippocampus were protected by C. asiatica extracts. The levels of catalase, superoxide dismutase, and lipid peroxidase in the hippocampus and striatum were improved indicating a neuroprotective property of the extract. Additionally, the effect of C. asiatica on cognitive function of healthy elderly volunteer was evaluated in a randomized, placebo-controlled; double-blind study involving 28 healthy elderly participants. The subjects have received the plant extract at various doses ranging from 250 to 500 and 750 mg once daily for 2 months, and cognitive performance and mood modulation were assessed.

It was found that high dose of the plant extract enhanced working memory and increased N100 component amplitude of event-related potential. Improvements of self-rated mood were also found following the C. asiatica treatment. The high dose of C. asiatica used in the study was suggested to increase calmness and alertness after 1 and 2 months of treatment. However, the precise mechanism(s) underlying these effects still require further investigation.

Catharanthus roseus (Madagascar periwinkle) is a well-known medicinal plant that has its root from the African continent. The interest in this species arises from its therapeutic role, as it is the source of the anticancer alkaloids vincristine and vinblastine, whose complexity renders them impossible to be synthesized in the laboratory; the leaves of this species are still, today, the only source. C. roseus originates from Madagascar but now has a wide distribution throughout the tropics, and the story on the traditional utilization of this plant can be retraced to Madagascar where healers have been using it extensively to treat panoply of ailments.

It is commonly used in traditional medicine as a bitter tonic, galactogogue, and emetic. Application for treatment of rheumatism, skin disorders, and venereal diseases has also been reported. roseus has been found to contain a plethora of phytochemicals (as many as 130 constituents) and the principal component is vindoline (up to 0.5%).

The oral administration of water-soluble fractions and ethanolic extracts of the leaves have been found to show significant dose-dependent reduction in the blood sugar at 4 h by 26.2, 31.4, 35.6, and 33.4%, respectively, in normal rats. In addition, oral administration of 500 mg/kg 3.5 h before oral glucose tolerance test (10 mg/kg) and 72 h after STZ administration (50 mg/kg IP) in rats showed significant antihyperglycaemic effects. No gross behavioural changes and toxic effects were observed up to 4 mg/kg IP.

Extract at dose of 500 mg/kg given orally for 7 and 15 days showed 48.6 and 57.6% hypoglycemic activity, respectively. Prior treatment at the same dose for 30 days provided complete protection against streptozotocin (STZ) challenge (75 mg/kg/i.p. × 1). Enzymatic activities of glycogen synthase, glucose 6-phosphate-dehydrogenase, succinate dehydrogenase, and malate dehydrogenase were decreased in liver of diabetic animals in comparison to normal ones and were significantly improved after treatment with extract at dose of 500 mg/kg p.o. for 7 days. Results indicate increased metabolization of glucose in treated rats. Increased levels of lipid peroxidation measured as 2-thiobarbituric acid reactive substances indicative of oxidative stress in diabetic rats were also normalized by treatment with the extract.

Vincristine and Vinblastine are antimitotic as they bind to tubulin and prevent the formation of microtubules that assist in the formation of the mitotic spindle; in this way, they block mitosis in the metaphase. These alkaloids are highly toxic; they both have neurotoxic activity (especially vincristine) because the microtubule assembly also plays a role in neurotransmission. Their peripheral neurotoxic effects are neuralgia, myalgia, paresthesia, loss of the tendon reflexes, depression, and headache, and their central neurotoxic effects are convulsive episodes and respiratory difficulties. Other side effects are multiple and include alopecia, gastrointestinal distress including constipation, ulcerations of the mouth, amenorrhea, and azoospermia.

Recently, new phenolic in different plant parts (leaves, stems, seeds, and petals), including flavonoids and phenolic acids, were reported. In addition, a phytochemical study concerning several classes of metabolites was performed and bioactivity was assessed. The high antioxidant potential of C. roseus was demonstrated in vitro using the radicals DPPH, superoxide, and nitric oxide.

Cyclopia genistoides is an indigenous herbal tea to South Africa and considered as a health food. Traditionally, the leafy shoots and flowers were fermented and dried to prepare tea. It has also been used since early times for its direct positive effects on the urinary system and is valued as a stomachic that aids weak digestion without affecting the heart. It is a drink that is mainly used as a tea substitute because it contains no harmful substances such as caffeine. It is one of the few indigenous South African plants that made the transition from the wild to a commercial product during the past 100 years. Research activities during the past 20 years have been geared towards propagation, production, genetic improvement; processing, composition, and the potential for value adding.

A decoction of honeybush was used as a restorative and as an expectorant in chronic catarrh and pulmonary tuberculosis. Drinking an infusion of honeybush apparently also increases the appetite, but no indication is given of the specific species. According to Marloth, honeybush was praised by many colonists as being wholesome, valuing it as a stomachic that aids weak digestion without producing any serious stimulating effects on the heart. It also alleviates heartburn and nausea. Anecdotal evidence suggests that it stimulates milk production in breast-feeding women and treats colic in babies.

Modern use of honeybush is prepared as an infusion and at times taken together with rooibos. The tea bags usually contain a larger percentage of rooibos than honeybush. Parts of other indigenous South African plants and fruits mixed with honeybush include dried buchu leaves, pieces of African potato (Hypoxis hemerocallidea) corms, and dried marula (Sclerocarya birrea) fruit. The ready-to-drink honeybush iced tea market is not developed to the same extent as that of rooibos, while honeybush "espresso," amongst others, has not been tried.

Honeybush is well known as caffeine-free, low tannin, aromatic herbal tea with a wealth of polyphenolic compounds associated with its health-promoting properties. The exact biologically active phytochemicals from honeybush are unknown, but the beneficial effects have been justified based on phenolic compounds. The major compounds, present in all species analyzed to date, are the xanthones, mangiferin and isomangiferin, and the flavanone, hesperidin.

Recently, two benzophenone derivatives 3-C-β-glucosides of maclurin and iriflophenone were isolated for the first time from C. genistoides and were tested for pro-apoptotic activity toward synovial fibroblasts isolated from rheumatoid arthritis patients. The strongest proapoptotic activity was obtained for isomangiferin and iriflophenone 3-C-β-glucoside, which were not previously evaluated as potential antiarthritic agents. Proapoptotic effects were recorded for mangiferin and hesperidin, which are major polyphenols in all commercially used honeybush plants. Recently, C. genistoides has attracted much attention for the production of an antioxidant product high in mangiferin content. The latter and its sustainability make C. genistoides an attractive source of mangiferin. Other potential applications are for the prevention of skin cancer, alleviation of menopausal symptoms, and lowering of blood glucose levels.

Harpagophytum procumbens is native to the red sand areas in the Transvaal of South Africa, Botswana, and Namibia. It has spread throughout the Kalahari and Savannah desert regions. The indigenous San and Khoi peoples of Southern Africa have used Devil's Claw medicinally for centuries, if not millennia. Harpagophytum procumbens has an ancient history of multiple indigenous uses and is one of the most highly commercialized indigenous traditional medicines from Africa, with bulk exports mainly to Europe where it is made into a large number of health products such as teas, tablets, capsules, and topical gels and patches.

Traditional uses recorded include allergies, analgesia, anorexia, antiarrhythmic, antidiabetic, antiphlogistic, antipyretic, appetite stimulant, arteriosclerosis, bitter tonic, blood diseases, boils (topical), childbirth difficulties, choler etic, diuretic, climacteric (change of life) problems, dysmenorrhea, dyspepsia, edema, fever, fibromyalgia, fibrosis's, gastrointestinal disorders, headache, heartburn, indigestion, liver and gall bladder tonic, malaria, migraines, myalgia, neuralgia, nicotine poisoning, sedative, skin cancer (topical), skin ulcers (topical), sores (topical), tendonitis, urinary tract infections, and vulnerary for skin injuries. The major clinical uses for Devil's claw are as an anti-inflammatory and analgesic in joint diseases, back pain, and headache. Evidence from scientific studies in animals and humans has resulted in widespread use of standardized Devil's claw as a mild analgesic for joint pain in Europe.

Chemical constituents according to the published literature include potentially (co)active chemical constituents: iridoid glycosides (2.2% total weight) harpagoside (0.5–1.6%), 8-p-coumaroylharpagide, 8-feruloyl-harpagide, 8-cinnamoylmyoporoside, pagoside, acteoside, isoacteoside, 6′-O-acetylacteoside, 2,6-diacetylacteoside, cinnamic acid, caffeic acid, procumbide, and procumboside. The constituent 6-acetylacteoside, being present in H. procumbens and absent in H. zeyheri, allows users to distinguish between the two species. Other compounds include flavonoids, fatty acids, aromatic acids, harpagoquinone, stigmasterol, beta-sitosterol, triterpenes, sugars (over 50%), and gum resins. Harpagoside isolated from H. procumbens varies within the plant and is the highest in the secondary tubers, with lower levels in the primary roots. The flowers, stems, and leaves appear to be devoid of active compounds. Iridoid glycosides isolated from H. procumbens tend to show dose-dependent anti-inflammatory and analgesic effects equivalent to phenylbutazone; they are apparently inactivated by gastric acids. Harpagoside is the most effective when given parenterally and loses potency markedly when given by mouth; enteric coated preparations might maintain efficacy despite exposure to gastric acids. Harpagoside has also been reported to inhibit arachidonic acid metabolism through both cyclooxygenase and lipoxygenase pathways.

There are varying and contradictory opinions regarding the anti-inflammatory and analgesic effects of Devil's claw in the treatment of arthritic diseases and low back pain. The controversy revolves around the active constituent of Devil's claw and its mechanism of action, as it appears to be different than that of nonsteroidal anti-inflammatory drugs (NSAID). The evidence from scientific studies in animals and humans has resulted in widespread use of standardized Devil's claw as a mild analgesic for joint pain in Europe.

Several clinical studies have been performed to determine the effectiveness of H. procumbens for its use as anti-inflammatory, general analgesic (commonly for lower back pain), and anti-rheumatic agent. To determine the effectiveness on lower back pain, Harpagophytum extract

WS1351 was administered in two daily doses of 600 and 1200 mg containing 50 and 100 mg of harpagoside, respectively, and compared to placebo. This randomized double-blind study took place over 4 weeks and subjects () with chronic susceptibility to back pain and current exacerbations with intense pain were included. Out of 183 subjects that completed the trial, six in the 600 mg and 10 in the 1200 mg were reported "pain-free" without using Tramadol (rescue pain medication). However, data analyses suggested that the 600 mg group reaped more benefits where less severe pain and no radiation or neurological deficit was present. The patients with more severe pain tended to use more Tramadol but not to the maximum permitted dose.

Momordica charantia, also known as bitter melon, is a tropical vegetable grown throughout Africa. The leaf may be made into a tea called "cerassie," and the juice, extracted from the various plant parts (fruit pulp, seeds, leaves, and whole plant), is very common folklore remedy for diabetes. charantia has a long history of use as a folklore hypoglycemic agent where the plant extract has been referred to as vegetable insulin.

Several active compounds have been isolated from M. charantia, and some mechanistic studies have been done.

Khanna et al have reported the isolation from fruits, seeds, and tissue culture of seedlings, of "polypeptide-p," a 17-amino acid, 166-residue polypeptide which did not cross-react in an immunoassay for bovine insulin. GA lactose binding lectin with a molecular weight of 124,000 isolated from the seeds of M. charantia has been evaluated for its antilipolytic and lipogenic activities in isolated rat adipocytes and found comparable to insulin. Extracts of fruit pulp, seed, leaves, and whole plant of M. charantia have shown hypoglycemic effect in various animal models. Karunanayake et al.found a significant improvement in glucose tolerance and hyperglycemia when the fruit juice of bitter melon was administered orally to rats. Fresh as well as freeze-dried M. charantia was found to improve glucose tolerance significantly in normal rats and noninsulin dependent diabetics (NIDDM) [105–108]. It was hypothesized that M. charantia fruit contains more than one type of hypoglycemic component. These may include an active principle called "charantin," a homogenous mixture of β-sitosterol-glucoside and 2-5-stigmatadien-3-β-ol-glucoside that can produce a hypoglycemic effect in normal rabbits.

A study administered the ethanolic extract of the fruit of bitter melon to STZ diabetic rats orally at a dose equivalent to 200 mg extract per kg body weight. Ninety minutes after the administration, they found that blood glucose levels had been reduced by 22%. The glycogenic enzymes-glucose-6-phosphatase and fructose 1, 6-bisphosphatase in the liver were also depressed. Further evidence for a beneficial chronic effect is that an improvement in both glucose tolerance and fasting blood glucose levels was observed in 8 NIDDM patients following 7 weeks of daily consumption of powered M. charantia fruit. Although some authors have indicated that the effect of M. charantia is not associated with an increase in circulating insulin, Welihinda et eland Welihinda and Karunanayake demonstrated that an aqueous extract from the fruit of M. charantia was a potent stimulator of insulin release from β-cell-rich pancreatic islets isolated from obese-hyperglycemic mice. Recently, Matsuura et al. have isolated a α-glycosidase inhibitor from M. charantia seeds which can be a potential drug therapy for postprandial hyperglycemia (PPHG).

However, Dubey et al. found that the aqueous, methanolic, and saline extracts of M. charantia produced a significant hypoglycemic effect in rats. In addition, the methanol and saline extracts also prevented adrenaline-induced hyperglycaemia.

When tested on laboratory animals, bitter melon has shown hypoglycaemic as well as antihyperglycaemic activities. Polypeptide-p isolated from fruit, seeds, and tissue of bitter melon showed potent hypoglycaemic effects when administered subcutaneously to gerbils, langurs, and humans. The aqueous extracts of M. charantia improved oral glucose tolerance test (OGTT) after 8 h in normal mice and reduced hyperglycaemia by 50% after 5 h in STZ diabetic mice. In addition, chronic oral administration of extract to normal mice for 13 days improved OGTT while no significant effect was seen on plasma insulin levels. We recently reported that M. charantia fruit extracts have a direct impact on transport of glucose in vitro.

Pelargonium sidoides is native to the coastal regions of South Africa, and available ethnobotanical information shows that the tuberous P. sidoides is an important traditional medicine with a rich ethnobotanical history.

P. sidoides root extract EPs 7630, also known as Umckaloabo, is a herbal remedy thought to be effective in the treatment of acute respiratory infections. There are numerous studies about P. sidoides and respiratory tract infections. These studies showed that P. sidoides may be effective in alleviating symptoms of acute rhinosinusitis and the common cold in adults, but doubt exists. It may be effective in relieving symptoms of acute bronchitis in adults and children and sinusitis in adults. EPs 7630 significantly reduced bronchitis symptom scores in patients with acute bronchitis by day 7. No serious adverse events were reported. EPs 7630 have a positive effect on phagocytosis, oxidative burst, and intracellular killing of cells. P. sidoides extract modulates the production of secretory immunoglobulin an in saliva, both interleukin-15 and interleukin-6 in serum, and interleukin-15 in the nasal mucosa.

In one research, P. sidoides was documented to represent an effective treatment against common cold. It was reported to significantly reduce the severity of symptoms and shortens the duration of the common cold compared with placebo. Because of these effects, the authors have aimed at establishing whether or not P. sidoides could affect the asthma attack frequency after upper respiratory tract viral infection. Results for some 20 clinical trials have been published, 7 of which were observational studies and the remaining 13 were randomized, double-blind, and placebo-controlled. For 6 of those 13 trials, only preliminary results have been published. All trials have been carried out using EPs 7630 in liquid or solid forms.

Medicinal plants are an integral part of the African healthcare system since time immemorial. Interest in traditional medicine can be explained by the fact that it is a fundamental part of the culture of the people who use it and also due to the economic challenge: on one side, the pharmaceutical drugs are not accessible to the poor and on the other side, the richness and diversity of the fauna and flora of Africa are an inexhaustible source of therapies for panoply of ailments . Nonetheless, there is still a paucity of clinical evidence to show that they are effective and safe for humans. Without this information, users of traditional medicinal plants in Africa and elsewhere remain skeptical about the value of such therapies. This denies people the freedom to choose plants that are potentially less costly and are more accessible. Another issue concerning the use of botanical remedies is the need to understand the safety of these therapies. For these reasons, information about efficacy and safety of traditional medicines is urgently required. The present paper has endeavored to overview just a few common medicinal plants from the African continents which have short- as well as long-term potential to be developed as future phytopharmaceuticals to treat and/or manage panoply of infectious and chronic conditions. Within the framework of enhancing the significance of traditional African medicinal plants, aspects such as traditional use, phytochemical composition, and in vitro, in vivo, and clinical studies pertaining to the use of these plants have been explored.

During the last few decades, it has become evident that there exists a plethora of plants with medicinal potential and it is increasingly being accepted that the African traditional medicinal plants might offer potential template molecules in the drug discovery process. Many of the plants presented here show very promising medicinal properties thus warranting further clinical investigations. Nonetheless, only few of them have robust scientific and clinical proofs and with a significant niche market (e.g., Aloe ferox, Artemisia afra, Aspalathus linearis, Centella asiatica, and Pelargonium sidoides) and a lot more have yet to be explored and proved before reaching the global market.

In the light of modern science, significant efforts should be geared to identify and characterize the bioactive constituents from these plants. Indeed, the discovery of therapeutic compounds from traditional medicinal plant remedies remains a medically and potentially challenging task. For adventure in such an attempt, highly reproducible and robust innovative bioassays are needed in view of our limited understanding of the multifactorial pathogenicity of diseases. Innovative strategies to improve the process of plant collection are needed, especially with the legal and political issues surrounding benefit-sharing agreements. Since drug discovery from medicinal plants has traditionally been so time-consuming, it is also of uttermost importance for investigators to embark and devise new automated bioassays with special emphasis on high throughput procedures that can screen, isolate, and process data from an array of phytochemicals within shorter time lapse for product development. Additionally, these procedures should also attempt to rule out false positive hits and dereplication methods to remove nuisance compounds.

Nonetheless, despite continuous comprehensive and mechanism-orientated evaluation of medicinal plants from the African flora, there is still a dearth of literature coming from the last decade's investigations addressing procedures to be adopted for quality assurance, authentication, and standardization of crude plant products. Appropriate standardization could be achieved via proper management of raw material, extraction procedures, and final product formulation. Without effective quality control, consistency and market value of the herbal product may be compromised. Indeed, one of the main constraints to the growth of a modern African phytomedicine industry has also been identified as the lack of proper validation of traditional knowledge and also the lack of technical specifications and quality control standards. This makes it extremely difficult for buyers, whether national or international, to evaluate the safety and efficacy of plants and extracts, or compare batches of products from different places or from year to year. This is in marked contrast with Europe and Asia where traditional methods and formulations have been recorded and evaluated both at the local and national levels. This would also tend to justify why the level of trade of phytomedicines in Asia and Europe is blooming more than those in Africa.

It is also imperative that potential risk factors, for example, the contamination of medicinal plant products with heavy metals from African traditional medicine products, be addressed and that regulatory guidelines are not only carefully developed but also enforced. Controlled growth (under GACP) and processing environments (under Good Manufacturing Practice) need to ensure that contamination of medicinal plant material is kept to a minimum. For the medicinal plant industry, cultivated plant material is preferred as it is easier to control the supply chain plus contamination is nominal. On the other hand, proper identification of a medicinal plant material is fundamental to the quality control process; it must be established unmistakably that the source of the plant material is genuine. Following this, microbial contamination (fungal, bacterial, and any potential human pathogens) must be checked during the stages of processing of the material. Chemical, pharmacological, and toxicological evaluations, conducted according to the principles of Good Laboratory Practices (GLPs), will certify the bioactive properties of the material undergoing processing.

These tests also are often the predictors of safety of the products manufactured. Clinical safety and efficacy will need to be established through exhaustive and usually lengthy trials during the early stages of the development of a therapeutic agent. After that, so long as the standard operating procedures are adhered to, then the unit dosage forms produced will be considered safe. Notwithstanding this, quality assurance procedures must be instituted so that the products coming from the factory are of good quality, safety, and efficacy.

To this effect, during the development stage, product standardization, quality control and assurance, double-blind, placebo-controlled, and randomized clinical controlled trials using standardized products or products containing pure plant extracts are essential components that need to be perfected in order to translate the potential of African botanicals into a reality for human to benefit.

4. The Importance of alternative medicine

The answer to the latter part of this question is undoubtedly "yes" and they are often more efficient and less harmful than many conventional drug therapies. Some of our old herbs and remedies, which served for hundreds of years, are now enjoying a renaissance, with growing ranges of natural medicines for both people and animals. However, time constraints in our fast-paced lifestyles make more conventional medicines an easy choice. Not only do pharmaceuticals sometimes take effect faster than natural alternatives (not necessarily curing, but masking the symptoms), but the average first consultation for Alternative Medical treatment lasts about 60-90 minutes, compared with the more usual 10 or 15 minutes conventional approach. Unfortunately, this often results in alternative treatments being used as a last resort, when in fact they are a valuable first line of treatment.

It worries me that, as humans, we are so quick to go to the doctor or chemist to receive medication for the littlest of things, when a gentler and more appropriate form of treatment, in proportion to the severity of the symptoms, will often suffice. We should be leaving the "big guns" where they belong, which is to fight the acute wars in life threatening situations.

So many drug resistances (especially antibiotics), are caused by indiscriminate use of the potent bug killers for the minutest of infections. It is only a matter of time before the so-called MRS (multiple resistant strain) infections - those hospital-based super bugs that no known antimicrobial agent is able to kill – are found in our daily environments.

As members of the medical profession, it is our duty to help prevent this from happening. But at the same time, as members of the public, it is our duty not to railroad the medical profession into using the big guns for our minimal diseases. Society has conditioned us to believe that it is unacceptable to take the necessary time off for our body's own immune system to sort the minor problem out, where in fact, this is exactly what we need to be doing for optimal health and longevity.

Conventional drug therapy often holds no parallel when it comes to acute, life threatening conditions. It certainly has a very important part to play in modifying disease processes too. Used over a short term, these pharmaceuticals carry a lower risk of drug induced side effects. However, long term use of pharmaceutical medication in chronic inflammatory, degenerative or cancerous conditions, is designed on the whole to help manage the condition by masking its symptoms. Very rarely does it lead to a cure of the disease.

Over time, more and more of the pharmaceutical drug is required and the chances of side effects become greater. Quite often, additional drugs are required to counter the side effects of the first ones. On the contrary, complementary and alternative medicines have a very good reputation for modifying chronic inflammatory and degenerative disease toward either complete cure or at least slowing down the development of the disease processes without dramatic side effects.

What is the role of complementary and alternative health care and medical practices in the health and well-being of the public? With this extraordinary collection of articles and essays, the Journal explores this question and helps to open a new period in the history of public health. Although long an integral part of the health systems of societies all around the globe, the relationship between public health and traditional or indigenous health practices has not often been a congenial or collegial one. Yet the question of the proper role of complementary and alternative medicine

(CAM) in the health of the public remains perhaps the most important one to be asked by readers of the Journal, both supporters and detractors of approaches that are beyond the pale of conventional biomedicine. It is a question with a complex set of answers.

First, it is critical that policymakers and public health personnel gain an understanding of the extent to which complementary and alternative health care forms an integral, albeit often marginal or marginalized, part of the public health apparatus at the disposal of any society. CAM may represent a substantial and largely untapped resource base. The World Health Organization estimates that most people in developing nations receive the bulk of their health care from traditional or indigenous health systems.

In Mozambique, for example, where there is one physician for every 50 000 people, there is a traditional healer for every 200. However, this is not a phenomenon of underdevelopment. Estimates for the United States, the United Kingdom, and Australia all hover near the 50% mark as well, and in France, 75% of the population report the use of alternative medicines.

In terms of control over social, scientific, political, and economic discourses, what some scholars call "biomedicine" has held clear ascendancy in the United States for over a century. Indeed, it is biomedicine to which CAM is "complementary" or "alternative"—the National Center for Complementary and Alternative Medicine of the National Institutes of Health defines CAM as "those healthcare and medical practices that are not currently an integral part of conventional medicine."

As with so much of the American cultural scene, however, the health care system in the United States has been and remains a pluralistic, oft tempest-tossed sea teeming with dynamically evolving species of healing systems. We have only recently begun to take account of the contributions of this alternative and complementary sector to public health. In a recent reprise of Kerr White's classic 1961 study of the ecology of medical care, Green and colleagues4reported in The New England Journal of Medicine that complementary and alternative health care providers now account for 65 visits monthly per 1000 population, the overwhelming majority of which are paid out-of-pocket. This compares with 113 visits per 1000 to see a primary care clinician. The authors' narrow definition excluded other CAM activities such as self-care practices and home remedies.

The articles in this issue represent a wide range of therapeutic approaches. The National Institutes of Health classifies the major domains of CAM as "alternative medical systems," "mind-body interventions," "biological-based therapies," "manipulative and body-based methods," and "energy therapies." Alternative medical systems are complete systems of theory and practice that have evolved wholly or largely independently of conventional biomedicine. These include Indian ayurvedic medicine, traditional Chinese medicine, homeopathy, and naturopathy. Mind–body interventions are "designed to facilitate the mind's capacity to affect bodily function and systems."

These include conventional approach such as patient education as well as approaches considered complementary or alternative such as hypnosis or prayer. Biological-based therapies include herbal therapies, dietary supplements, dietary approaches, and the use of other biologically active substances. Manipulative and body-based methods include manipulation, movement, massage, or similar approaches, often within the context of physical or anatomic theories of illness. Finally, energy therapies focus on the role of energy fields within the body or from other sources in the production of disease and the process of healing.

This system of classification is one of several that have been proposed. However, the intellectual point of departure, and the standards by which these therapies are judged, remains that of conventional biomedicine.

A second consideration in addressing the role of CAM in public health is determining effectiveness and efficacy. Merely hosting a special issue on the topic of complementary and alternative public health will not magically resolve the thorny issues that have plagued debate in this area for the past several years. However, to shy away from this debate may be profoundly debilitating to public health in the long term. The complex ontological and epistemological issues involved strike to the very core of our "scientific" approaches to public health, and our ability to avoid conceptual stagnation and continue to gain new knowledge. There can be no question that social and political considerations of established biomedicine have often masqueraded as "scientific" just as surely as there have been charlatans or others blindly supporting untenable beliefs and practices at the expense of the public health.

An interesting compromise was reached in Germany with the passage of the German Drug Act in the 1970s. Concerned by the very idea that "science" could be used to prejudice judgment against potentially effective treatments led to the expansion of the very idea of what is scientific. Or rather, it could be argued that the German approach marked a return to the term's more inclusive meaning as a system of knowledge, and not necessarily the one and only received system of knowledge held by a biomedical scientific establishment. Perhaps from the land that gave the world Martin Luther, one should expect nothing less. The compromise solution involved alternative criteria for the proof of the effect and effectiveness of herbal drugs apart from randomized clinical trial data. In effect, the "scientific standard" by which the efficacy of herbal drugs could be assessed could now be other rational systems and models in addition to the ethno medical system known as biomedicine.

The cultural diversity of complementary and alternative health practices and systems can indeed be daunting. Kleinman[6] suggests that we understand a society's health care resources as belonging to 3 sectors: popular, folk, and professional. For public health practice and research, there is much to be gained in understanding these health sectors, including scientific biomedicine, as ethnomedical systems within society. Baer[7] has suggested that the American landscape is best understood as a pluralistic continuum of alternative or complementary ethnomedical systems.

This continuum ranges from professionalized biomedicine and the parallel medical system of osteopathy to professionalized heterodox systems such as chiropractic, acupuncture, and naturopathy to national and regional folk healing systems such as Appalachian folk medicine to self-care and home remedies used outside of these professionalized and semi professionalized systems. While, for instance, Native American health systems are easily understood to fall into a separate system of ethnomedicine, it is indeed helpful to understand that movements such as Christian Science, chiropractic, and spiritualism may also be indigenous ethnomedical systems in the United States.

This type of framework not only leads to interesting social, political, and economic questions but also helps us to understand that the tapestry of care resources for public health is indeed rich. Such a broad reconceptualization of the public health system offers many potential opportunities to improve, expand, and refine what we do, where we do it, for whom we do it, and to what end. This is as true in the developing world, such as in western Africa, as it is in the industrial world, such as in the American South. The opportunity to increase the power and reach of the public health sector through integration of CAM or indigenous practitioners is ignored only at our own detriment.

One final consideration must be raised. The past (and present) insensitivity of public health workers and scientists to complementary, alternative, or indigenous systems of health may, at best, reflect a long history of arrogance, exploitation, and colonialism.[10]At worst, it represents a continuing legacy of intellectual, emotional, and spiritual violence committed in the name of the very public we have sworn to protect. Can one claim that a society is healthy that finds its worldview under automatic assault, and the integrity of its culture called into question? This is not a call for cultural relativism so much as a call for cultural tolerance and humility. We may, indeed, have much to learn from one another.

How may we decide on the health of a culture itself? This has been a vexing theoretical and pragmatic question confronting anthropology since Henry Lewis Morgan essentially founded the discipline in the 19th century by trying to salvage what he saw as the disappearing culture of the Iroquois. Healthy societies are composed of healthy individuals, but they are not simply the sum of these parts. Nor can the health of individuals be maximized in the context of ailing social systems or cultures. What role does public health play in promoting and maintaining the health of societies and cultures, particularly in the era of globalization?

Whether it is an integrated model of holistic health care for Native American women, the role of the Black churches in the South in providing mental health services,[9] or drawing upon the lessons of shamanic healing in providing brief psychotherapy for Latino immigrants, the works collected in this special issue represent a snapshot of complementary and alternative approaches that can play a vital role in the health of the public.

Although the standard of positivist biomedical science may not always be a fair point of departure, it is nonetheless the framework within which we decide truth. It can be a purely reductionist model of scientific reason, with its linear model of causality and attempts at objectivity. It can also be a less reductionist approach, where causality may be understood more as a web rather than a thread, and the subjectivity of lived experience once again assumes a prominent role in understanding health and well-being. With this less reductionist approach, the interrelationships between cultural and personal, public and individual health begin to become clearer.

The works collected here represent the beginning of an important dialog for public health. Although in different ways, complementary and alternative health care and healing practices represent a vast and as yet unrealized sector of the public health systems of developed and developing nations. Moreover, the limits of our current biomedical knowledge and capabilities cannot be denied. We do not, as yet, have all the answers, or even, for that matter, know all the questions. There are more things in heaven and earth than can be dreamt of in our current biomedical philosophies. Stagnant biomedical orthodoxy cannot achieve the fullness of public health's potential and has no role to play in human progress. Maintaining openness to this reality may serve to help marshal the resources of indigenous, complementary, and alternative health practices in the service of public health, now and in the future.

Alternative medicine is a practice of consuming a medicine without the use of drugs. Alternative medicine has a number of benefits. It is a practice of consuming a medicine without the use of drugs. This may involve herbal medicines, self-awareness, biofeedback, or acupuncture.

With alternative medicines, a person becomes an active participant in techniques involved in the cure. Individuals understand their physical body functions well and understand the way it relates to their health. Holistic medicine comes under alternative medicine. Nature, as a whole, has an important role in the usage of fruits, herbs, detox, and vitamins for purification, stimulation and healing. Use of such therapies has gained popularity in recent times, since they offer great health benefits to users. Many people are directing their attention toward alternative medicine and natural therapies for prevention of illnesses and solving their day-to-day health-related issues.

Benefits and Usage of alternative medicine

The natural therapies present in alternative medicines are age-old as compared to western form of treatments such as antibiotics and surgeries. According to physicians, most alternative medicine therapies started with clinical impressions or scientific research. The medicines are safe and involve natural substances. One primary objective of alternative medicines is to relieve people from depending largely on drug usage and help them manage their lives naturally. For users' convenience, below given are some ways to use alternative medicines:

- People following an alternative medicine may do physical exercises such as osteopathy, yoga; infuse physical activity, tai chi, meditation and reflexology. To do these exercises, place the pillow on a surface providing comfort to the body, since these exercises stimulate and manipulate structural balance of the body. In addition, the exercises improve overall bodily functions. Users may practice these exercises for mental, physical, spiritual and emotional benefits.

- Users may undergo massage therapy, which involves manipulating and rubbing the body tissue for mental and physical relaxation. They may do this either at home or at a massage clinic. When at home, apply massage oils to the neck, forehead, feet and hands.

- Change the way of thinking. Exercise the mind first, so the body follows it. Meditate for relaxing the mind, thinking positively and clearing stress. Take deep breaths for better healing. Simultaneously, make use of enhanced visualization of objects for forming good thought patterns.

- For relaxing the body, drink herbal teas. Improvement of bodily functions depends on what people eat and drink, since the same relieves, stimulates and has a healing effect on the body. Consume fresh fruits, vegetables and vitamins daily so that the body gets essential nutrients. Drink ginger tea since it is effective in the cure of nausea and heals the body naturally.

-Those who wish to develop strong bones and healthy muscles may seek the help of a chiropractor. Chiropractic is a method of treatment that manipulates the body structures, especially the spine to relieve low back pain or even headache or high blood pressure. The chiropractor shows people their pressure points.

- A simple, yet curable method that comes under alternative therapy is laughter as being the best medicine. People have experienced miraculous changes in certain health disorders due to mere laughing. As such, it is advisable people watch comedy shows on TV. Read magazines and books that promote laughter. Alternately, cleanse the entire body with essential oils, herbs, fruits that have certain therapeutic benefits on the skin. Combine herbs, natural products and fruits together as a remedy to skin disorders.

- Users may try alternative medicines such as the electromagnetic therapy and biofeedback, which controls body functions such as heart rate, brain activity and blood pressure. People have turned to using alternative medicine, since it offers multiple health benefits and cures them from long-term ailments in a natural way.

Alternative or complementary methods of care are being used in hospitals and clinics in growing numbers. Alternative methods are a significant and important support to healing and, I think, should definitely be included in your agenda. The awareness and accepted validity of complementary/alternative medicine is part of transforming the culture of medicine right along with taking a participatory role. There is no mention of Alternative/Complementary Care on the JoPM website, nor is there any topic for it in the call for papers. Since the mission of the Journal of Participatory Medicine is to transform the culture of medicine to be more participatory–with an invitation to participate to create a robust journal to empower and connect patients, caregivers, and health professionals–it makes sense that complementary medicine should be included, since so many people use it. While it remains true in medicine that most patients have been trained by our culture to depend upon the doctor to know what is best for them (and thus the reason for the participatory medicine movement), as you know, the growing trend is for patients/clients to take responsibility for their own care in a collaborative effort with caregivers. But we need to take it a step further. Patients/clients need to understand the importance of taking responsibility for themselves on all levels, not just physically, but emotionally, mentally, and spiritually. It's time to acknowledge that human beings are one integrated being, and to go beyond the common "lip service" given to "holistic" in medicine. This includes the undeniable fact that all parts/aspects of a human being affect all other parts/aspects. We are much more than the sum of our parts.

One last thought about alternative care…the same idea of depending upon a practitioner or doctor in medicine also carries into alternatives or complements to medicine. The possible benefits of using alternative medicine as self-directed care are largely unknown, even among its proponents, and require education about how to use it in this way. But before education can begin, acceptance of its validity is essential. Whether alternatives are used through a practitioner or in self-directed care, I believe that awareness of their importance should be known. Thus, alternative/complementary care has a place in this work your journal is doing to transform the culture of medicine.

There are several reasons why it is imperative to add alternative medicine to your healthcare arsenal. The focus of holistic and self-awareness healing has been shown to bridge the gap for certain shortcomings of modern Western medicine.

Traditional healthcare or Western medicine has been used in the United States and Western Europe for the past two centuries. It is defined as medical treatment based on the use of drugs and surgery to treat symptoms (signs of illness).

Western medicine has been criticized for its reliance on drugs to treat symptoms of an ailment as opposed to treating the root of the problem. The lack of any holistic approach to total body health as you know is a great cause for concern. In the past decade, Western medicine has finally caught-on and begun adopting certain alternative medicine concepts.

One of my approaches to healthcare is to incorporate a holistic approach that treats the entire body instead of focusing on a single body part or symptom. Healthcare is so much more than just medicine it involves all aspects of mental, physical, emotional, and spiritual health.

To give you a little bit of background, alternative medicine covers a broad range of treatment. It is often referred to as complimentary alternative medicine (CAM) because it is used along with traditional medicine practices. The emphasis is on education, prevention, and holistic treatment.

Practices commonly used include acupuncture, aromatherapy, Chinese medicine, chiropractic, herbal medicine, homeopathy, massage, meditation, therapeutic touch, and yoga.

There are several reasons why alternative medicine is a powerful and crucial addition to modern healthcare. Alternative medicine allows you to participate and take responsibility for your health – providing more options when seeking a treatment that fits their needs.

You'll find alternative medicine recognizes stress and lifestyle choices that can negatively affect health. Proper nutrition, exercise, rest, and emotional balance have been proven to have a heavy impact on physiological well-being. All these aspects and much more are taken into consideration when diagnosing health problems.

Practices like yoga and acupuncture may have been used for centuries but have only been scientifically researched in the last several decades. Interest in holistic treatments has increased with scientific evidence proving efficacy.

Many physicians are now realizing what I realized long ago – and now regularly recommend certain alternative medicine practices to treat blood pressure, chronic pain, depression, and anxiety.

Yoga and meditation have been shown to decrease blood pressure and improve immune function. For example: turmeric can eliminate chronic pain and this ancient spice has been proven effective in alleviating some of the worst symptoms of Alzheimer's disease. Massage and chiropractic care also help manage chronic pain without drugs.

Another importance of alternative medicine is its power to eliminate the use and abuse of over-the-counter (OTC) medication. Regular use of common pain relievers such as Tylenol™ can cause liver damage, stomach ulcers, and increase your risk of stroke.

Certain herbal medicines should not be taken with prescribed medications or during pregnancy. Always consult your healthcare practitioner before attempting an alternative medicine therapy. They will know if a certain alternative medicine is safe to use with your current treatments.

Alternative medicine offers a great alternative option for treatment modalities when used safely. I urge you to make alternative treatment a part of your daily healthcare and find out all about my latest breakthroughs and discoveries.

5. Traditional Medicine vs. Alternative Medicine

In modern Western culture, we have become accustomed to thinking of "traditional" medicine as what is practiced in mainstream doctors" offices and hospitals. Natural or alternative medicine, by contrast, takes a holistic approach to treatment, looking at the overall person and the whole body, rather than simply the symptoms being experienced. In many cases, natural medicine works on preventing the body from becoming ill or depleted. Meanwhile, conventional medicine, in which treatments are based on the results of scientific trials, tends to treat the symptoms that patients experience, as well as some diseases. However, generally speaking, conventional medicine looks at these symptoms in isolation and usually after the illness has already occurred. Conventional medicine is also known as allopathic medicine or Western medicine. The name Western medicine came about because many of the alternative therapies and natural healing practices currently in use originate from the East. What is Alternative Medicine? Although it is called alternative, traditional medicine is widely used around the world. In fact, in many countries, herbal medicines are given before conventional medical treatment. Alternative medicine has always been popular in developing countries, and its popularity in industrialized nations is increasing rapidly. In India, the alternative medicines were known as Vedic medicines or Aired. Ayurveda has been practiced for thousands and thousands of years and is still in practice. The aim of Ayurveda medicine is balancing the harmony of mind, soul and body. Ayurveda is an alternative medicine made from herbs, certain vegetables, fruits and natural minerals. There are historical evidences that surgeries were also performed as part of ayurveda treatment in olden days.

Ayurveda prescribes alternative medicines for curing common cold, stroke and paralysis and certain mental diseases. In China, alternative medicine was practiced for centuries and its concept is based on Taoist philosophy. The practice of alternative medicine in China that also spread to Japan and Korea is known as Oriental branch of alternative medicine. The two schools that contributed to the practice of alternative medicine and therapies are "Jinfang" and "Wenbing". You must be aware of the term "acupuncture". This originated in China and is used to treat various orthopedic and neurological ailments and is popular even today. Chinese treated the human mind and the body and not the disease. They believed a strong human body could never fall sick. Uses of Traditional Medicine Most people are familiar with the tools of conventional medicine, such as blood tests and x-rays, but what exactly does natural medicine entail? Traditional medicine may use plant-, animal- and mineral-based products for treatment. It may also include spiritual and manual therapies. Some types of alternative therapies include: acupressure: massage in specific areas for pain relief.

Acupuncture: the insertion of thin, heated needles into the body to treat symptoms and balance the energy Chinese herbal medicine: the use of plant-based remedies to treat or prevent illness. Energy therapies: the practice of channeling energy through the hands for healing. (Reiki is a type of energy therapy.) Homeopathy: the use of small amounts of natural remedies to treat illness. Kinesiology: the use of muscle tests to identify and correct imbalances in the body. Massage therapy: the practice of manipulating skin, muscles and joints to relieve stress and pain. Eastern Medicine versus Western Medicine Debate about the merits of Eastern medicine versus Western medicine (also referred to as natural vs. allopathic medicine) has been going on for years. Arguments against the use of natural medicine focus on the lack of verifiable scientific data that proves it works. Although studies have been done on traditional Eastern medicine, many of these have been criticized for not being rigorous enough. Others have focused on the fact that the results of studies receive negative press, even when they appear to work for the target group most at risk. Other criticism focuses on the fact that people may take longer to seek conventional treatments. Instead, many people turn to natural medicines first, making it harder to achieve success with Western medicine. Issues relating to unwanted side effects of natural medicines, plus the fact that this area is virtually unregulated, are other reasons for concern. Finally, many alternative therapies are not covered by health insurance. In the end, only the patient can decide what treatment works best for them. The important thing is that the patient seeks treatment, either natural or conventional, and that the treatment heals. Acupuncture is another way of alternative medicine that has gained lots of popularity in United States.

Our culture has allowed the health care industry to become so powerful and disproportionately lucrative that it is now in the business of illness rather than health. In one disconcerting example, a cancer physician, returning from an extended vacation, found an empty waiting room. His colleague had been treating his patients nutritionally. The physician wailed, "This is terrible. It took me years to build a long-term, regular patient clientele!" People everywhere are realizing that our doctors receive no reward for health, only for treating illness.

Most medical schools don't teach disease prevention, proper diet or exercise as a part of health. Objective measures are emphasized - white blood cell counts, blood pressure readings, etc., instead of how the patient feels. Pain is treated as a powerful enemy, its symptoms assaulted with prescription drugs that mask it or drive it underground- a practice that usually means it will resurface later with increased intensity.

The twenty-first century finds many people using more natural, less drug-oriented therapies, sometimes as an alternative to conventional medicine, sometimes in a team approach along with it. As orthodox medicine becomes more invasive, and less in touch with the person who is ill, informed people are becoming more willing to take a measure of responsibility for their own health.

Health is a lifestyle process. It is based in wellness care, instead of just illness treatment. The best news is that natural remedies work - often better than prescription drugs for many health conditions.

Orthodox medicine focuses on crisis intervention and is less successful in treating chronic illness. Many modern medical techniques were developed during war time, for emergency care. However, respected studies show that most illnesses don't just drop out of the sky and hit us over the head. Arthritis, osteoporosis, lower back pain, high blood pressure, coronary-artery disease and hormone imbalances are related to aging and lifestyle. The emergency measures tend to overkill, and even suppress the body's own immune response. Mental anxiety is brought on by needless testing, medication, or treatment, and a brusque or rushed doctor. You can literally worry yourself sick when there is nothing seriously wrong.

Our culture has allowed the health care industry to become so powerful and disproportionately lucrative that it is now in the business of illness rather than health. In one disconcerting example, a cancer physician, returning from an extended vacation, found an empty waiting room. His colleague had been treating his patients nutritionally. The physician wailed, "This is terrible. It took me years to build a long-term, regular patient clientele!" People everywhere are realizing that our doctors receive no reward for health, only for treating illness.

Most medical schools don't teach disease prevention, proper diet or exercise as a part of health. Objective measures are emphasized – white blood cell counts, blood pressure readings, etc., instead of how the patient feels. Pain is treated as a powerful enemy, its symptoms assaulted with prescription drugs that mask it or drive it underground- a practice that usually means it will resurface later with increased intensity.

The twenty-first century finds many people using more natural, less drug-oriented therapies, sometimes as an alternative to conventional medicine, sometimes in a team approach along with it. As orthodox medicine becomes more invasive, and less in touch with the person who is ill, informed people are becoming more willing to take a measure of responsibility for their own health.

Many modern medical techniques were developed during war time, for emergency care. However, respected studies show that most illnesses don't just drop out of the sky and hit us over the head. Arthritis, osteoporosis, lower back pain, high blood pressure, coronary-artery disease and hormone imbalances are related to aging and lifestyle. The emergency measures tend to overkill, and even suppress the body's own immune response. Mental anxiety is brought on by needless testing, medication, or treatment, and a brusque or rushed doctor. You can literally worry yourself sick when there is nothing seriously wrong.

The human body is a beautifully designed healing system that can meet most problems without outside intervention. Even when outside help is needed, healing is enhanced if the patient can be free of emotional devastation, depression and panic. Emotional trauma impairs immune function and panic constricts blood vessels, putting additional burden on the heart.

Alternative healers recognize that pain is also the body's way of informing us that we are doing something wrong, not necessarily that something is wrong. Pain can tell us that we are smoking too much, eating too much, or eating the wrong things. It can notify us when there is too much emotional congestion in our lives, or too much daily stress. Pain can be a friend with useful information about our health, so that we can effectively address the cause of the problem.

Not every problem requires costly, major medical attention. Healthy food, regular moderate exercise and restful sleep are still the best medicine for many health conditions. The principle of nature governing health and illness are ageless; they apply equally everywhere at all times. There is no down time with the laws of nature, and they do not play favorites.We need to be re-educated about our health – to be less intimidated by doctors and disease. I believe that the greatest ally of alternative medicine will be science itself – not the restricted view of science that assumes its basic concepts are complete, but the open-ended science that sets preconceived notions aside. Today's consumers are not only more aware of alternative health care choices and more confident in their own healing strength, but also want to do something for them to get better. The time has clearly come for a partnership between health care professionals and patients, so that the healing resources from both sides can be optimally employed.

The dictionary states that conventional medicine is offered by hospitals and practiced by those who have a medical doctor degree; it is also called western medicine. The opposite of conventional medicine is called complementary and alternative medicine (CAM). Complementary and Alternative medicine can be considered holistic medicine, which is usually not prescribed by physicians a part of hospitals. There has been an increase in those that have an aversion to conventional medicine that is offered by hospitals (Astin, 1998). There are multiple reasons as to why people dislike conventional medicine. Some reasons for this increase are that "alternative treatments are thought to offer more control over health care.

Other common complementary and alternative treatments can include; acupuncture, chiropractors, yoga, tai chi and homeopathies (Eisenberg, 1997). Since CAM treatments were all that were known back in the day, they were considered godsends. However, in the fourteenth and fifteenth centuries the witch trials began. These trials changed the belief that CAM treatments were good until recent times (Alsleben and Donsbach, 1992). The respect of CAM treatments was lost during the witch trials because all those that were thought of as being witches used herbal medicine and in general complementary and alternative medicine. The history of conventional medical treatments started after complementary and alternative medical treatments stopped being respected (Alsleben and Donsbach, 1992). It is believed, that conventional treatments branched off of CAM treatments because of when they started being in use. There is some research or knowledge about complementary and alternative medical treatments; however, more needs to be done. More research needs to be done so that a plethora of different people can make wise decisions. It is known that most CAM treatments are used for allergies.

Conventional medicine is traditional medicine that the majority of us are familiar with — local doctors, clinics, hospitals, pharmacies. It's the kind of medicine the average physician practices. Alternative medicine includes a philosophy and practice that is inclusive of a variety of world cultures.

When it comes to medicine and treatment, we often live in a bubble, thinking that traditional medicine is the only way. Because of global communication and the openness of the internet, however, more and more people are becoming aware that there are alternatives to traditional medicines.

Some doctors are strictly traditional practitioners, others are strictly alternative, but some practice both together.

The main difference between traditional medicine and alternative medicine is the approach. Whereas traditional medicine treats symptoms and problems of a certain given area, alternative medicine focuses on cause and prevention, overall health, and non-traditional, often natural treatments.

There are a variety of alternative medicines: Osteopath, herbal medicine, massage, acupuncture, homeopath, chiropractic. Some people are hesitant to try alternative medicine, but this is because our society has been bred from the start to suspect anything different from the status quo, or that hasn't been approved by the FDA.

We are slowly emerging from the dark ages when it comes to embracing alternative ways to stay healthy. Alternative medicine isn't less effective or less reliable — sometimes it works when nothing else will — it's simply misunderstood, and those that question it are likely to be uninformed or misinformed. Alternative medicine is widely accepted and used throughout the world. The US is beginning to catch up.One advantage to alternative medicine is cost. It's less expensive to seek and to use natural or alternative remedies. But you should ask yourself, why does medicine have to be expensive to work?

Many employers offer healthcare packages with alternative medicine. The trend to seek alternative treatments is growing. Many alternative products can be found on shelves next to traditional medicines.

When it comes to traditional medicine, symptoms are addressed with drugs or surgery. If your liver is giving you trouble, it's your liver that becomes the focus, not the entire body. Think of all the specialists who focus on one organ of the body. A cardiologist focuses on the heart. A neurologist focuses on the brain. A lung specialist focuses on the lungs. With all the focus being in one area, one can see why traditional medicine sometimes falls short in addressing the entire health of the patient. Traditional medicine is based on research, lab experiments, and trials.

While this is the accepted approach, it may not be the best approach for the individual. Individuals have individual needs that traditional medicine may not address.

6. Reasons for using CAM

It is important to understand the reasons why people use CAM. Generally, illness is associated with a convergence of the biological, psychological, and social factors. However, conventional medicine, with its focus on the biological causes of disease, is not sufficient to acknowledge the interrelatedness of mind, body and spirit that is essential to holistic care. The reasons for CAM use are not limited to biological disequilibrium; psychological and social-cultural factors can also influence a patient's decision and preference to use CAM. The next section of this review explores the physical, psychological, and therapeutic benefits, and the social-cultural and traditional aspects shaping the rapidly growing use of CAM. Available literature exploring the reasons, perceived benefits and clinical efficacy experienced by users of CAM with a mental disorder is somewhat limited, but suggests that people use CAM because of their value and belief system and perceived benefits from CAM.

Russinova et al. (2002) found that 86% of individuals seemed to benefit from a variety of alternative medicines. Astin, Pelletier, Marie and

Haskell (2000) also indicated that 80% of elderly persons had received substantial benefit from their use of CAM. Alternative medicine enhanced their social, spiritual, general 49 and self-functioning. Perceived benefits have been identified as important factors influencing the decision to use alternative medicine for various health problems (Astin, 1998). There appear to be a number of reasons associated with CAM use. These reasons can be categorized as: 1) health promotion and disease prevention, 2) immune system benefits, 3) increased energy, 4) ideological, cultural and philosophical congruence, 5) clinical efficacy and success, symptom relief, 6) health characteristics, 7) recognition of the limitations of conventional medicine, and 8) criticism of conventional medicine. Health promotion and disease prevention Health promotion and disease prevention have been identified as important factors that can influence a person's attitudes toward the use of CAM (Astin, 1998).

Yamashita et al. (2002) reported that half the Japanese respondents (n = 760) showed a high expectation of health promotion or disease prevention from CAM. Japanese people purchased nutritional drinks and dietary supplements to maintain or promote optimal health. General health promotion is also the most popular reason for using such therapies among older people (Astin et al., 2000; Lewis et al., 2001). Immune system benefits CAM is also often used to improve the immune system. Whilst depression is a complex, multifactorial disease whose etiology has not yet been fully elucidated, it has historically been treated with medication, psychotherapy or electro convulsive therapy (ECT). Although the biological mechanisms by which depression alters the endocrine and nervous systems are not yet clear, there is evidence that depression may alter immune responses (Herbert & Cohen, 1993).

High pressure stress was found to induce immunosuppression. Some forms of CAM may have effects on the immune system. Evidence suggests that the application of citrus fragrance, which stimulates the olfactory system, markedly reduces the dose of antidepressants necessary for treatment (Komori et al., 1995). Neuroendocrine hormone levels and immune function could be normalized by treatment with citrus fragrance. 50 Increased energy Fatigue is an important somatic symptom of depression. Depressed persons are more prone to fatigue (Hayslip, Kennelly, & Maloy, 1990; Skapinakis, Lewis, & Mavreas, 2003).

In a secondary analysis of the World Health Organization Collaborative Project on Psychological Problems in General Health Care conducted by Skapinakis, Lewis and Mavreas (2003), a total of 5,438 primary care patients from 14 countries were assessed with the Composite International Diagnostic Interview. They reported that patients with depression or anxiety were more likely to report unexplained fatigue. Several studies have identified a positive association between CAM use and an intention to increase energy or diminish fatigue (Astin, 1998; Astin et al., 2000; Baldwin et al., 2002; Eisenberg et al., 1998). Rickhi, Quan, Moritz, Stuart and Arboleda-Flórez (2003) conducted a study in Canada to compare patients with and without mental disorders who seek services from complementary therapy practitioners. They found that 26.6% of patients with a mental disorder saw a complementary practitioner for fatigue.

The mind-body-spirit interconnections are the essence of CAM holistic belief systems (Astin, 1998; Barry, 1996; Dossey, Keegan, Guzzetta, & Kolkmeier, 1995). The concept of holism, which refers to the belief that health is harmonizing the body, mind and spirit, is associated with positive attitudes toward alternative medicine (Astin, 1998; Siahpush, 1998). People use CAM because of their belief in the importance of treating the whole person and focusing on the connection of body-mind-spirit (Lewis et al., 2001). Breda and Schulze (1998) argued that advances in medical technology often fail to heal the whole person. In other words, the biomedical treatment model cannot adequately incorporate the specific beliefs and influences of psychological, psychosocial and spiritual factors on health. The reasons why people in different countries seek CAM needs to be understood. The question of whether culture, beliefs, and traditions contribute to CAM use or the meaning of illness is integral to effective and holistic healthcare delivery. Moreover, knowledge of culture and people's health beliefs allows health professionals to 51 communicate more effectively and formulate culturally sensitive care plans. A number of studies have attempted to relate the expressed preferences for CAM with socio-cultural considerations, tradition and beliefs.

Astin (1998) conducted a survey on the reasons why people use alternative medicine in an attempt to develop models to explain their use. The study revealed that culture is a powerful factor in influencing the use of alternative therapy. 'Cultural creative' is a significant predictor of use, and is described by Astin as being those who have beliefs and are committed to a range of values and beliefs about the nature of life, spirituality and the worldview, or who have philosophical orientations. The nature of health and illness may be understood in very different ways in different cultures (Astin et al., 2000). Ethnic or racial backgrounds will colour choices and responses to such therapy. The use of CAM is thus tightly connected and influenced by cultural paradigms. Charlton (1993) added that the context of spirituality and life meaning may be an important factor in attracting consumers of CAM to treat their illnesses. Religious beliefs and attitudes may influence the use of CAM. Mitzdorf et al. (1999) reported that 50% of CAM users had supportive religious beliefs. Moreover, 79% believed that CAM would help their suffering and 76% believed that CAM practitioners could succeed when others couldn't.

These results suggest that strong beliefs and socio-cultural factors impact on the use of CAM. A supportive family environment has also been reported to have a positive effect on CAM use (Divertie, 2002). Family members' awareness, opinions and attitudes towards the patient's illness are connected to CAM use. Clinical efficacy and success, symptom relief some forms of CAM are reported to be effective even though the exact physical mechanism is unknown. The response of getting relief for symptoms, diminishing pain or discomfort, and feeling better suggest that perceived benefits and clinical efficacy are potential determinants of CAM use. For example, in Eisenberg et al.'s (2001) study, respondents believed CAM therapies to be more helpful than 52 conventional cares for the treatment of headache and neck and back conditions. Conversely, people also judged that conventional medicine was more helpful than CAM for treatment of hypertension. The disease process can involve the most intense pain a patient will experience.

Fishbain, Cutler, Rosomoff and Rosomoff (1997), in a systematic literature review, investigated the association between chronic pain and depression. The experience of pain can lead to a sense of helplessness and has been associated with the subsequent development of anxiety and depression. Astin et al (2000) found that pain management was one reason why older people use CAM. Mitzdorf et al. (1999) also estimated that more than half of the respondents reported previous success using CAM for pain relief. Around 80% of respondents reported previous success from CAM in treating not only the symptoms, but also the causes of pain. CAM practitioners were reported to offer better and adequate advice for their patients to improve lifestyle, quality of life and nutrition.

Recognition of the limitations of conventional medicine While conventional medicine may be necessary for most health problems, there are some definite limitations, including side effects and other negative effects leading to 53 physical discomfort and increased resistance to conventional medicine. People may be frustrated by the obvious limitations of conventional medicine. As Singh, Raidoo and Harries (2004) indicated, for 37.6% of CAM users, modern (conventional) medicine led to an improvement in symptoms, but was unable to treat the underlying medical conditions. Lam (2001) explored the strengths and weaknesses of traditional Chinese medicine and conventional medicine and found the majority of participants recognised that traditional Chinese medicine and conventional medicine each have strengths and weaknesses. Traditional Chinese medicine is considered as being good for curing the underlying cause or root of the disease or disorder. Seeking to address the advantages and disadvantages of both health services, participants reported that they do not solely rely on traditional Chinese medicines for a health condition that conventional medicine can manage better, and do not seek help or treatment from conventional medicine for a condition that traditional Chinese medicines can manage or treat better. Participants also believed that each one should be utilized where it is more likely to be helpful. They therefore use conventional medicine to control the symptoms for faster recovery first, and then use traditional Chinese medicines to "completely cure the disease" (Lam, 2001). Furthermore, one of the strongest perceived advantages of traditional Chinese medicines is that they have very few side effects in comparison to conventional medicine, which has significant and negative side effects associated with its use.

Similarly, Yamashita, Tsukayama and Sugishita (2002) and Knaudt, Connor, Weisler, Churchill and Davidson (1999) reported that CAM therapies such as dietary and nutritional supplements appear to have no extremely harmful side effects at doses that are large enough to improve health problems. Significant side effects, for example the anticholinergic side effects of antidepressant medication (Luo, Meng, Jia, & Zhao, 1998), may be one of the main reasons that people turn to CAM, and this may influence their medication adherence to conventional medicine. Criticism of conventional medicine previous research has suggested that dissatisfaction with conventional medicine was an important factor in the growing popularity of CAM. Mitzdorf et al. (1999) indicated that two thirds of respondents had previous experiences or frustration with conventional medicine; more than 70% of respondents complained about the lack of success with previous treatments; and more than 80% complained about side effects of conventional drugs.

Similarly, in an exploratory study of an alternative therapy user group and a community sample in Australia, McGregor and Peay (1996) reported that those who choose to use alternative medicine had negative attitudes toward biomedicine and lacked confidence in the effectiveness of medical care. Lloyd, Lupton, Wiesner and Hasleton (1993) in a cross sectional survey of 289 patients from eight Sydney practices providing a range of alternative modalities, reported that those who used alternative therapies were mindful of pharmaceuticals; 31% expressed preferences for 'drug-free' treatment' and 41% were more satisfied with their interaction with CAM practitioners.

Yamashita et al. (2002) also found that CAM consumers (n = 760) reported a number of the negative aspects of conventional therapies such as dissatisfactory results (19.2%), and adverse or harmful side effects (17.1%). Astin et al. (2000) examined predictors of CAM use among 728 people over 65 years of age in the USA. They found that dissatisfaction with conventional therapy and fears of drug side effects were associated with CAM use. CAM's attraction emerges from these core reasons. Research exploring the reasons for CAM use among older people is limited. No study specifically focused on the reasons for using CAM among hospitalized patients diagnosed with depression.

7. Measures of CAM use

A list of twenty-four different kinds of CAM based on the work of Kessler et al. (2001) was also used in this study. It was assumed that as the categories were already established and no problems identified that the same list could be used and this would enable the opportunity for comparison of data. The following sections outline the areas surveyed during data collection. These included the following five sections: (1) CAM use, (2) reasons for use, (3) health care providers of CAM, (4) communication with health professionals about CAM use, and (5) support for CAM use (see Appendix B). CAM use The first question asked if participants had ever used any of the CAM listed in the past 12 months (Phase 1) and was coded as 0 = "no" or 1 = "yes". This question was also repeated when assessing CAM use one month following discharge (Phase 2), as different seasons or months of data collection may produce quite different results.

The collection of CAM data at two phases (when hospitalized and one month following discharge) increased the ability to produce consecutive estimations for CAM use over time and reliable estimations of CAM use for a population of people with depression. Harris and Rees (2000) support this premise and indicate that reliable and influencing factors are best explored over time. Although it might be expected that hospitalised, depressed patients may have difficulties remembering and/or concentrating, this issue was noted by the researcher and was effectively diminished by the continuous observation and discussion with patients' primary health care providers before collecting any data. The best time to approach potential participants for data collection was decided by patients' primary health care providers, based on patients' physical and mental conditions

The 24 CAM listed were also classified into four categories or domains as outlined by Kessler et al. (2001): cognitive feedback (relaxation techniques, imagery, self-help group, hypnosis, biofeedback); oral medicine (herbal medicine, megavitamins, 84 homeopathy, naturopathy); physical treatments (massage, chiropractics, osteopathy, acupuncture, yoga); and other therapies (spiritual healing by others, dietary modifications, lifestyle diet, special diet for losing or gaining weight, energy healing, aromatherapy, laughter, other therapy to treat pain, other lifestyle intervention programs and folk remedies). Reasons for CAM use Three questions were included on the reasons for CAM use. Participants were asked to indicate if they have ever used any of the 24 listed CAM for their depression and the reasons for their CAM use. Reasons were coded into six categories that were based on the work of Dougherty, Touger-Decker and Maillet (1999): disease prevention, immune system benefits, increased energy, improved feeling of wellbeing, symptom relief and disease treatment. Participants may report using more than one type of therapy and more than one reason for the type of therapy.

Participants also reported the frequency of CAM use in the past 12 months. Categories of frequency of use included once in a while, monthly, weekly and daily. Health care providers of CAM Participants were also asked about CAM health care providers. They were asked if they had ever seen any complementary or alternative care provider (yes/no). If yes, they were asked about the person who provided their CAM. Licensed therapists have received formal training and may be certified by a licensing board or related professional associations. For example, in Taiwan a doctor of Chinese medicine has usually received formal training in medical school, been awarded a degree and is licensed by the government. Licensed therapists are knowledgeable about specific CAM therapies and provide care or health advice about their use and usually receive payment for services from Medicare or consumers. Licensed therapists were categorised and included: general practitioner (GP), hospital professional therapist, private CAM clinic, and private CAM therapist. Unlicensed therapists are persons without appropriate education, training, credentials and competency.

A person practicing CAM prior to licensure is also considered an unlicensed therapist. 85 Communication with health professionals about CAM use two items were developed about communication with health professionals in regard to CAM use. Participants were asked if they had ever discussed their CAM use for depression with their psychiatrists and nurses (yes/no) respectively. Support for CAM use Support is known to influence therapy decisions and choice of alternative therapies (Baldwin et al., 2002; Lee, Charn, Chew, & Ng, 2004; Montbriand, 1993; Williamson, Fletcher, & Dawson, 2003) and assist people to cope with difficulties and challenges. In this regard, the situation for patients with a diagnosis of depression is no different from others who are dealing with significant treatment decisions. Participants were asked to indicate any person(s) who supported their use of CAM, for each CAM they had previously used.

The current study also aimed to identify factors associated with CAM use in the treatment of depression, for example, attitudes and perceived education about CAM by nurses. An exploration of the influence of CAM use on adherence to antidepressant medication was also addressed in the current study. A number of instruments were used and are outlined below.

For assessing adherence to antidepressant medication, participants were asked if they had used antidepressants in the 12 months prior to their current hospitalization. Information about this one-year prevalence of antidepressant use was coded as 0 = no or 1 = yes. This question was also repeated to assess prevalence of antidepressant use one month following discharge. 86 Attitudes toward CAM Individual's attitude may be important to determine one's acceptance of treatment. Ajzen and Fishbein also stated "attitudes could explain human actions". Attitude reflects how one feels about treatment. There has been little research on attitudes toward CAM as a contributing factor of CAM use among patients with mental illness in general, and depression, in particular. Although very few studies have attempted to investigate the relationship between attitudes toward CAM and CAM use among persons with mental disorders, the need for assessment of patient attitudes has been identified as an important factor in understanding how patients' seek help. Thus, in order to determine attitudes toward CAM in depressed patients, a scale was developed by the researcher (see Appendix D). This scale was developed using information from the review of several CAM studies and related literature.

Attitudes were assessed through sixteen items on 5-point Likert scales of 1 = strongly disagree to 5 = strongly agree. The questionnaire of attitudes toward CAM focuses on self-reported knowledge level, clinical efficacy for depression treatment and the issues related to a combination use of CAM and antidepressant medication. The critical aspects of harmfulness and helpfulness of CAM use were included in attitude assessment. Availability and cost are also common concerns related to attitudes toward CAM. Participants were asked about their intention to try CAM therapies since intention is the immediate determinant of health behavior (Pender, Murdaugh, & Parsons, 2002). If a person believed that CAM could be beneficial, he or she may be influenced to use CAM and remain adherent. Attitudes influence behavior indirectly through intentions (Fredericks & Dossett, 1983; Kahle & Berman, 1979).

Attitudes toward antidepressants this tool attempted to find out participants' attitudes toward antidepressants (see Appendix F). This brief tool, which originally measured the effects of physician communication style on client medication beliefs and adherence to antidepressant treatment, is part of a comprehensive inventory developed by Bultman and Svarstad (2000). The tool has been used previously to assess client medication beliefs among 87 100 participants who were prescribed antidepressants (Bultman & Svarstad, 2000). The questionnaire has six items and was developed using concepts from the Health Belief Model (HBM). Items 1 – 2 are positively phrased and 3 – 6 are negatively phrased. Participants indicate to what extent they agree with the statements on a 5-point Likert scale of 1 = strongly disagree and 5 = strongly agree. The scores for medication belief items were summed, with a possible range of 6 – 30. High scores are associated with more positive beliefs on the use of antidepressants.

Cronbach's alpha test for internal consistency of this scale was 0.65 (Bultman & Svarstad, 2000). Patient education about CAM An instrument was sought that would assist with an understanding of how patients perceived that nurses were involved in their education and decision about CAM use. As no suitable instrument was found an adapation of an existing instrument (Bultman & Svarstad, 2000) was required. Items developed by Bultman and Svarstad (2000) were based on concepts from the Health Communication Model (HCM) (Svarstad, 1986) and previous communication studies. In the original questionnaire, the items assessed the extent to which the physician's initial communication style encouraged client participation in the treatment process and were scored on a 4-point scale ranging from 0 = not at all to 3 = very much. Alpha coefficients for the instrument were 0.73 and suggested that the scale had acceptable internal consistency (Bultman & Svarstad, 2000). This scale was developed further by the researcher based on a review of the literature to fit the purpose of the current research (see Appendix E).

Additional features, such as the extent to which patients received education about CAM, were also measured. Although this scale was originally designed for physicians, the researcher adapted it for nurses. An example of modification required was: 'physician asked if I had questions or concerns' which was replaced with 'my nurses asked if I had questions or concerns about CAM use for my depression'; and the question 'physician helped with concerns related to the use of medication' was changed to 'my nurses helped me with my concerns related to the use of CAM'. 'Physician was friendly during initial visit' was substituted with 'my nurse was knowledgeable during our discussion'. The context of this last question was changed 88 in order to capture how patients perceived nurses' knowledge. It was assumed that nurses need to be knowledgeable in order to know how CAM interacts with conventional medicine. Furthermore it was assumed that if nurses were perceived as knowledgeable that patients would feel confident with nurses' ability to assist and support their treatment and decisions about CAM.

Thus, the questions also focused on asking participants if nurses: asked if they had questions and concerns about CAM use for treating depression; helped them with their concerns related to CAM use; were knowledgeable about CAM during the discussion; gave them clear instructions on how to use CAM for depression; gave them clear explanations about how CAM would affect them; and talked about the types of CAM they could use to help them feel better. Finally, three items asked whether or not nurses listened to patients; gave written information about CAM; and whether a follow-up appointment was made when the nurse and patient finished their first discussion about CAM.

In order to maintain a uniform format, the responses were presented in a 5-point Likert scale format ranging from 1 = strongly disagree to 5 = strongly agree. The nine items were summed for a possible score range of 9 – 45. A high score is associated with more patient education. Patient education about antidepressants This questionnaire was originally designed by Lin et al. (1995) to assess whether patients received any of the 12 patient education messages from the primary care physician, and whether the physician discussed any of the six listed cognitive activities. For the purpose of this study, the researcher made modifications to 14 items of the Lin et al. questionnaire to seek information on participants' perceptions of health education about antidepressants received from nurses rather than physicians (see Appendix E).

For example, education about continuing to take antidepressants even if they felt better, side effects, noticeable effects, and taking antidepressants on a daily basis without interruption. Participants were asked to rate their agreement on a 5-point Likert scale of 1 = strongly disagree to 5 = strongly agree. The items were summed for a possible score range of 14 – 70. A high score is associated with nurses 89 giving more patient education about antidepressants. Given the high proportion of Taiwanese people taking CAM and the possibility of drug interaction with conventional medicine the researcher was interested in identifying through this scale whether nurses had included CAM education into their patient education role. Adherence Attitude Inventory to antidepressants The Adherence Attitude Inventory (AAI) (Lewis & Abell, 2002) was chosen for this study to ascertain adherence attitudes to antidepressant medication among this sample population. The AAI has not been widely used for the assessment of adherence attitudes in diverse clinical populations or with different cultural backgrounds. The authors claim that the AAI does not measure adherence to medication directly, but instead aims to measure four factors with well-known correlations to adherence: cognitive functioning, patient-provider communication, self-efficacy, and commitment to adherence.

The AAI is a 28 item rapid assessment instrument developed from several major health behavior theories, namely, the health beliefs model, health promotion model, reasoned action, and planned theory (see Appendix H). The first construct, cognitive functioning, is based on research that indicated that not all non-compliant people reject their medications, but rather may simply forget to take those (Lewis & Abell, 2002). The second construct, patient-provider communication, is based on the theory that effective communication increases the potential to explore patient opinions regarding possible barriers to medication adherence and patients' beliefs about their capacity to remain adherent. The third construct, self-efficacy, is based on the health promotion model, which emphasizes the importance of self-efficacy as a useful predictor of future performance in self-managing medication. The final construct within the AAI is commitment to adherence, which reflects the likelihood of an individual complying with a suggested treatment.

The survey contains 28 items. Participants were asked to indicate their response on a 5-point scale of 1 = none of the time to 5 = all of the time. The scores for all items were summed, with a possible range of 28 – 140. 90 Lewis and Abell (2002) used a number of methods to verify the validity and reliability of the AAI and found the instrument to be sound. Validity was evaluated using factor analysis to determine the accuracy of this instrument. Factor analysis assesses the degree to which the items within a scale truly cluster together and become one or more subscales (Bean land, Schneider, LoBiondo Wood, & Haber, 1999). The findings from the factor analysis indicated that the AAI has a strong factor structure (Lewis & Abell, 2002).

Furthermore, the authors were concerned with whether the items were representative of the content domain of geriatric mental health. Content validity was undertaken and submitted to an expert panel for review. The test of reliability and validity suggested that the AAI would be an efficient and effective research instrument for the current research. All instruments, except demographic data, were repeated one month following discharge to determine changes over time. The adherence attitude inventory was added in Phase 2. Thus, there were 82 questions in total at Phase 1 and 100 questions at Phase 2. The survey included a mix of both 5-point Likert scale and yes/no responses covering demographics, measures of severity of depressive symptoms, CAM use and measures of factors related to CAM use.

8. CAM Use by the General and rural People

In 2000, Stephen E. Straus, MD, Director of NCCAM, addressed the Senate Appropriations Subcommittee regarding budgets for the fiscal year 2001, asking for an increase of $3,381,000 above the fiscal year 2000 appropriation. The reason for this increase was growing public interest in CAM (NCCAM, 2003e). Ott (2002) suggests another reason for increased CAM use in her article on meditation in pediatric clinical practice—that CAM is used in addition to conventional medical treatment, complementing the patient's existing medical treatment.

Therefore, patients do not have to abandon their prescribed medical treatment. They can add to it, perhaps with a feeling that they are contributing to the healing process. Considering the concept of "complementing" brings greater understanding to results of the studies by Eisenberg et al. in 1993 and 1998, where a surprising number of participants reported CAM use. In the subsequent study, CAM use increased and was paid for out of pocket. Gordon et al. (1998) discovered that 25% of HMO members had recently used CAM and that 90% of adult primary care and obstetrics-gynecology physicians in the study had recommended one or more alternative therapies.

A large portion of the members surveyed from this same HMO (70%) desired CAM therapies to 29 be available to them in their plan. In that same study, physicians were found to favor HMO coverage for CAM therapies to complement behavioral medical treatments. Demographically, Eisenberg et al. (1993) found that most users of CAM were non-black, ranged from 25 to 49 years of age, were more educated, and had higher incomes.

Eighty-three percent had seen a medical doctor for chronic conditions and got no relief Seventy-two percent of these same respondents did not disclose CAM use to their conventional medical physicians. Ni, Simile, and Hardy (2002) found that of 30,801 adults queried (response rate 70%), CAM use was lower in men than in women (33.4% and 24.0%). Again, it was found that people with more education were more likely to use CAM.

People in the Midwest and West were more likely to use CAM than in the Northeast or South. Notably, 86.7% of CAM users had conventional medical primary care providers. Astin (1998) set out to study why people would choose CAM in the United States. Some of what Astin found validated what Eisenberg et al. (1993, 1998) discovered: Users of CAM were usually more educated. What compelled most study respondents to use CAM was not dissatisfaction with conventional medicine. The study found that the majority of CAM users feel that CAM is more congruent with their own philosophies, values, and beliefs regarding life and health (Astin, 1998). Additionally, most of the respondents who reported using CAM suffered from chronic health problems, such as back problems, allergies, and lung problems. This study, like the two done by Eisenberg et al. (1993, 1998), was not exclusive to any particular group or population.

One group of people that has recently emerged as the focus of studies regarding CAM is rural people. From a varied sample of rural, older adults residing in the Southeastern United States, one group of researchers found that most of the people sampled used a form of CAM, such as vitamin therapy, home remedies, faith, or herbs (Arcury, Quandt, Bell & Vitolins, 2002). Vallerand's research discovered that of urban, suburban, and rural patients in Michigan who suffered from pain, the rural residents were less likely to use CAM (Ham,

2003). Of the group, 77% of the urban and 82% of the suburban subjects used CAM in managing pain This contrasted with only 58% of the rural residents using CAM to assist in pain relief.

This may be because the suburbanites had higher incomes and could afford to pay out of pocket for CAM (which is usually not covered by insurance). Some of the highest levels of poverty in Michigan are in rural areas, so this could be a powerful influence on whether or not a rural person might use CAM (Fedstats, 2003). Research conducted by Johnson (1999) studied rural elderly women in the western United States.

The majority of the women had greater than 12 years of education and incomes of over $40,000 per year. Johnson's sample is probably not representative of most rural women, especially rural women in Montana. However, some of the findings are congruent with others' findings about traits of rural people (Lee, 1998). The women in Johnson's (1999) sample shared characteristics of rural people such as "selfsufficiency, independence, and the ability to care for themselves." Therefore, Johnson surmised that health care consultation and practices outside the established norm 31 appealed to their independent nature. They liked the independence of being able to manage self-care without the required prescription or office/clinic visit.

Appealing as well was the sense the women had of being in control and self-reliant with regard to their self-care, health promotion, and disease management. In spite of the characteristics of independence and self-reliance that rural people exhibit (Lee, 1998), cost can influence and alter decisions. The cost of CAM might influence a person to use CAM if prescribed medications were out of reach financially. On the other hand, a person might decide not to use CAM since out-of-pocket payment is required.

Level of education plays a major role in whether a subject uses CAM (Eisenberg et al., 1993; Astin, 1998). It also seems that people who have a holistic health philosophy are more likely to use CAM (Astin, 1998). In the study by Johnson (1999), the subjects chose CAM due to their self-reliance and independence. It also appears that having a chronic health condition is a predictor for CAM use (Astin, 1998; Eisenberg et al., 1998). In summary, the literature supports that use of CAM is present and appears to be increasing. However, little is known about rural people and CAM use, particularly rural people living in large, sparsely populated states like Montana.

9. Advantages and disadvantages of alternative medicine

In today's day and age we are recognizing more and more about the effects that our bodies are having with what we put inside of them. There are many advantages to using alternative medicine over the typical mainstream prescriptions and medicines. Health care professionals themselves are even becoming more and more open to alternative medicine and the benefits it can have for the body.

- It treats the Actual Cause. One of the best advantages that alternative medicine offers is that it heals the body and is designed to actually treat the cause of the pain or disease that has occurred. By understanding and treating the disease, Chiropractors and other alternative medicine professionals are able to work at the root of the problem. Mainstream medicine, on the other hand, tends to treat the symptom that the disease or pain is causing, not actually treating the cause.

-It is an improvement of the Quality of Life. When we use prescription drugs we generally see an improvement in pain, but once the drug goes out of our system the pain returns. When using alternative medicine, there is a drastic improvement in the quality of life a person has.

-It is safer. Alternative medicine is a wide spectrum of therapies, and they are almost always considered to be much safer than mainstream medicine. Natural remedies are used to correct the problem. There are no man-made, unnatural substances that you would be using to put in your body.

-It does not have bad side effects. When using mainstream medicine you might be able to get rid of your headache, but the side effects might include nausea, hallucinations and risk of stroke in the process. Almost all mainstream medicine has some type of warning about the bad side effects that come from taking it, where natural remedies don't.

-It is more flexible. Alternative medicine allows more flexibility in treatment plans. Many chiropractors and alternative medicine professionals' change their treatment plans according to lifestyle changes, where mainstream medical professionals wouldn't.

-It looks at overall health of your body. Alternative medicine focuses on healing pain and disease by balancing out other aspects of your life. Sleep, nutrition and stress can affect your body, so adapting health plans with these in mind is important with alternative medicine. Mainstream medicine is not nearly as well rounded.

-It doesn't offer dependency treatment options. Prescription pills can cause dependency and other harmful side effects to the body and mind. Alternative medicine does not have those same disadvantages.

The natural therapies present in alternative medicines are age-old as compared to western form of treatments such as antibiotics and surgeries. According to physicians, most alternative medicine therapies started with clinical impressions or scientific research. The medicines are safe and involve natural substances. One primary objective of alternative medicines is to relieve people from depending largely on drug usage and help them manage their lives naturally. For users' convenience, below given are some ways to use alternative medicines:

-People following an alternative medicine may do physical exercises such as osteopathy, yoga, infuse physical activity, tai chi, meditation and reflexology. To do these exercises, place the pillow on a surface providing comfort to the body, since these exercises stimulate and manipulate structural balance of the body.

In addition, the exercises improve overall bodily functions. Users may practice these exercises for mental, physical, spiritual and emotional benefits.

-Users may undergo massage therapy, which involves manipulating and rubbing the body tissue for mental and physical relaxation. They may do this either at home or at a massage clinic. When at home, apply massage oils to the neck, forehead, feet and hands.

-Change the way of thinking. Exercise the mind first, so the body follows it. Meditate for relaxing the mind, thinking positively and clearing stress. Take deep breaths for better healing. Simultaneously, make use of enhanced visualization of objects for forming good thought patterns.

-For relaxing the body, drink herbal teas. Improvement of bodily functions depends on what people eat and drink, since the same relieves, stimulates and has a healing effect on the body. Consume fresh fruits, vegetables and vitamins daily so that the body gets essential nutrients. Drink ginger tea since it is effective in the cure of nausea and heals the body naturally.

-Those who wish to develop strong bones and healthy muscles may seek the help of a chiropractor.

Chiropractic is a method of treatment that manipulates the body structures, especially the spine to relieve low back pain or even headache or high blood pressure. The chiropractor shows people their pressure points.

-A simple, yet curable method that comes under alternative therapy is laughter as being the best medicine. People have experienced miraculous changes in certain health disorders due to mere laughing. As such, it is advisable people watch comedy shows on TV. Read magazines and books that promote laughter. Alternately, cleanse the entire body with essential oils, herbs, fruits that have certain therapeutic benefits on the skin. Combine herbs, natural products and fruits together as a remedy to skin disorders.

-Users may try alternative medicines such as the electromagnetic therapy and biofeedback, which controls body functions such as heart rate, brain activity and blood pressure. People have turned to using alternative medicine, since it offers multiple health benefits and cures them from long-term ailments in a natural way.

According to Johns Hopkins University, more than 40 percent of Americans report using alternative medicine therapies for pain control when prescribed medications prove to be ineffective. Alternative medicine offers an integrated approach to healing and may include interventions such as herbal remedies, reflexology, chiropractic, nutritional supplements, massage therapy and acupuncture. With more medical professionals beginning to suggest the use of alternative therapies in combination with conventional medical treatments, many more studies are underway to examine both the usefulness and safety of these nonstandard treatments.

Pain

Many people turn to alternative medicine therapies for pain relief when traditional treatments fail to work. Alternative medicine also offers treatment options to individuals who do not have access to pain clinics under their health insurance plans. A study conducted by researchers at the University of Michigan Health System found that older individuals, who are more likely to suffer chronic pain conditions, use alternative therapies more frequently. Results of the study are published in the January 2010 issue of the journal Pain Medicine. The study takes a look at the increasing use of alternative treatment modalities as a way to manage chronic pain.

Cancer

Alternative medicine therapies used together with conventional medical treatments can alleviate some of the symptoms of cancer, as well as lessen the negative side effects of conventional medical treatments. Chemotherapy, although effective in increasing the survival rate of many cancer patients, can produce unpleasant side effects. Some cancer patients are able to tolerate chemotherapy treatments better when using an alternative treatment such as acupuncture to control side effects like fatigue, headache, nausea, vomiting, night sweats and aching.

Cost

Alternative medicine therapies can be less expensive than conventional medical treatments. Although some alternative therapies are not cheap, many herbal remedies and other natural treatments still cost less than prescription medications and treatments. Acupuncture and chiropractic sessions can cost significantly less than conventional pain therapy treatments.

Side Effects

In most cases, effective alternative therapies have fewer or no side effects as opposed to the frequent and sometimes severe effects of many prescription medications and other conventional medical treatments. But depending on what medical conditions a person might have, even natural remedies and other alternative therapies can sometimes cause adverse side effects. Not all natural remedies have been scientifically tested, nor does the FDA regulate them. Treatment modalities such as therapeutic massage and acupuncture are generally considered to be safe, but always talk to your doctor before using any alternative medicine therapies.

Mental Health

Alternative medicine can be beneficial to a person's overall wellbeing, as the approach focuses on healing the mind, body and spirit. Treatment methods such as massage therapy, biofeedback, meditation and visual imagery help a person to relax and reduce stress. Art and music therapies are used to relieve symptoms of depression and schizophrenia by stimulating the natural release of endorphins and opiates in the body, in addition to helping individuals let go of deeply repressed emotions. The Substance Abuse and Mental

Health Services Administration points out that other alternative approaches to mental health, such as diet and nutrition, animal-assisted therapies and self-help groups can be valuable resources for improving mental health.

Over the past few years' people have changed their attitude to conventional methods of treatment and more likely try alternative medicine. Is it only a new trend or maybe the most efficient manner to back on one's feet? Below I display some advantages and disadvantages of alternative therapy.

Herb treatment, acupuncture, homeopathy or aromatherapy – nowadays people are surrounded by these names and it's nothing new that someone leave traditional methods and replace them by unconventional ones. When all of conventional treatments disappointed us we are automatically searching for something new. First undeniable advantage of alternative medicine is the fact that it consist of a broad range of healing philosophies, approaches, and therapies. Thanks to this everyone can find something suitable for his ailment.

Furthermore, we can practice many of alternative methods of treatment in home and the cost of therapies is in many cases surprisingly low. For a basic set of herbs or oils to aromatherapy we pay not more than a few zlotys while modern specimens and remedies are very expensive and many people can't afford them.

On the other hand, although acupuncture and chiropractic fees are sometimes covered, most of alternative treatments are not reimbursed by health insurance, which is definitely one of disadvantages of this kind of medicine. Despite the fact that unconventional methods have many benefits as complements or alternatives to conventional therapies, these kinds of products and services are not without their risks to people. For example, improper use of herbal remedies can create a host of problems for older persons, who may have different responses to these products when compared with younger adults.

What is more, the current interest and enthusiasm directed towards alternative treatments is understandable, but the full risks and benefits of them are still unknown so we can't be sure about possible effects of therapy.

Taking everything into account there are many positive sides of alternative medicine, but unfortunately nothing is perfect.

- Targets the root cause. Most alternative and complementary medicine is used not only to treat the symptoms of the health condition but the root cause of it. Some of the procedures and remedies that are known for targeting the root cause of problems are acupuncture, herbs, massage, diet and exercise, and the like.

- The approach is holistic. Alternative medicine focuses on treating the whole person, not only the health condition. This means that whatever alternative remedy the practitioner's advice the patient to take is a customized approach to cater to all of the patient's physical, emotional, mental, and spiritual needs. This, according to the Osher Center for Integrative Medicine, may be why alternative and complementary medicine is making its way up.

- Pays personal attention. Imagine finding someone a gift, and not knowing so much about a person; most likely, you'll pick the wrong gift. In the same way, alternative medicine practitioners take time to know the patient more in order to better treat him/her.

- Emphasizes prevention. Conventional medicine is often focused on curing an existing problem while alternative and complementary medicine focus on prevention. Most practitioners persuade patients to have "well visits," scheduled appointments when the patient isn't sick.

- Reduces stress. Most alternative therapies reduce stress and emotional tension, helping to prevent or heal illnesses. Conventional medicine does not always prioritize this.

Ask a professional whether the alternative medicine is suitable for your health condition and lifestyle because the following are drawbacks of alternative medicine.

- Scientific research on alternative medicine is limited. Compared to conventional medical procedures, scientific research and studies on alternative medicine is still very limited. Funding for alternative medicine studies, however, are growing with the help of private sources. For the meantime, the National Center for Complementary and Alternative Medicine (NCCAM) advises that people ask health care providers or physicians, and visit the archives of NCCAM's research on their website.

- Confusion in marketing. When it comes to observing marketing campaigns, it's best to be a bit skeptical about it. Some health and wellness companies may use fillers or unrealistic taglines; oftentimes they say their products are natural when they are not necessarily all natural. It's best that the viewer or potential patient become more objective about these campaigns by keeping in mind that, just because the company says something is natural, doesn't mean it's entirely safe.

- Its best that the potential patient does his/her own research about the remedy or product he/she is planning to take. A few agencies' websites like the National Institutes of Health and the U.S. Food and Drug Administration may have information about it.

- Possible interference with prescription drugs. Some alternative medicine or herbs, despite not containing artificial substances, can still interact negatively with prescription drugs. The best way to find out if an alternative medicine will work for you is to ask for an opinion from a professional alternative medicine practitioner who is also a medical doctor.

Alternative medicine, alternative therapy, holistic therapy, and traditional medicine are some of the other names of complementary therapy. There are many kinds of treatments that exist under complementary therapy, and each has its own unique theory and practice. But to give it a general definition, complementary therapy is any type of medication, treatment, or technique that is not part of the modern, conventional medical system. Some of the most popular ones are aromatherapy, acupuncture, herbal medicine, and yoga.

It is becoming more common for people to use complementary therapies together with their conventional treatments because of the advantages alternative healing provides. Yet others remain skeptical and hesitant to try natural treatments because of their disadvantages.

They teach you to become more responsible for your health.

Holistic healing teaches you to regain the balance between your mind and body because the illnesses and pains that you feel are brought about by imbalances in your system. It focuses on helping you to pinpoint the root cause, and how to heal that root cause rather than just the symptoms. You will also learn how to maintain your overall wellness for long-term optimal health, so you become more empowered and proactive in taking care of your mind and body.

They may not be as costly as modern therapies and medications.

Some complementary therapies involve using only natural ingredients in medications and treatments, and these are usually readily available in your kitchen cabinet, your garden, or from your natural surroundings. Yoga, a popular alternative therapy, requires only a mat. Plus, you can do it almost anywhere without the need for special equipment.

They can work as sole, primary, or supportive treatments.

Recent studies show that certain herbs and foods help to control and heal cancer and diabetes. Those who have anxiety and depression also benefit from doing yoga and taking certain herbs according to certain tests. Therapeutic massage has been reported to also help relieve muscle and joint pain.

They take time to work. Most alternative treatments do not heal instantly. It usually takes several hours or even months before you can see any positive effects. This can be discouraging for some, especially if you have a nagging headache that you want to go away immediately. This is why some practitioners will not recommend complementary therapy for emergency situations.

They require lifestyle changes. You have to commit your time, energy, and sometimes even your finances if you really want to adopt holistic medicine as your method for gaining optimum health. This means having to make some major changes to your lifestyle, such as changing your diet and adopting a different mindset when it comes to dealing with the stressors in life. But if this leads you to improve overall well-being, then maybe this can be more of an advantage than a disadvantage.

They might interact with certain medication. Some herbal remedies might interact with prescription drugs, while some types of natural therapies might have contra-indications for your existing condition. That is why you must always inform your conventional or complementary practitioner about the medicines you are currently taking and the true status of your condition, and ask for their professional advice regarding incorporating alternative therapies for your healing.

More conventional medical practitioners are becoming more open to the use of complementary therapies as supportive treatments. However, you must still make sure that you make informed decisions before adopting any form of treatment, whether it is conventional or alternative.

10. Women's use of complementary and alternative medicine

This thesis draws upon the methods and principles of health services research to critically examine women's utilization of complementary and alternative medicine (CAM) during pregnancy. The epistemology of the thesis adopts a positivistic approach to knowledge, which is in line with applied health services research. This background chapter explores the role and value of health services research in the examination of all aspects of CAM utilisation and provides an overview of the structure of this thesis.

There is a danger of tying the CAM research programme exclusively to the issue of efficacy. In order to fully understand CAM we must broaden our approach beyond simply asking questions of clinical effectiveness, to include methods and research perspectives from neighboring traditions such as public 6 health, health services research and health social science.

Health services research examines how people get access to health care, the cost of healthcare, and what happens to patients as a result of this care (Horner, Russ-Sellers, & Youkey, 2013). It aims to identify the most efficient and effective approaches to healthcare delivery, management, organization and financing whilst maintaining patient centered care (Horner et al., 2013). The definition of health services research is ever evolving with the latest Academy Health (the professional organization of the health services research field in the USA) (Lohr & Steinwachs, 2002) definition stating: "Health services research is the multidisciplinary field of scientific investigation that studies how social factors, financing systems, organizational structures and processes, health technologies, and personal behaviors affect access to health care, the quality and cost of health care, and ultimately our health and well-being.

Its research domains are individuals, families, organizations, institutions, communities, and populations." This particular field of enquiry, health services research, was conceptualized in the early 1960s to study important healthcare issues such as cost, access, quality of care and patient outcome (Bindman, 2013) and since then, has evolved to become an integral part of the healthcare and medical research landscape. Investment in health services research helps to better plan for future health care in relation to the allocation of funding, setting appropriate healthcare priorities and the improved allocation of human and operational resources (Bindman, 2013; Adams, 2008).

Historically, health services research has focused upon conventional health care and very little has examined CAM. In the modern healthcare context though, CAM is popular, making up a significant component of health care/service utilisation. A health services research examination of CAM is vital to explore all facets of this utilisation. In order to completely characterize and understand CAM use it is crucial to expand the research gaze beyond randomized controlled trials designed to evaluate clinical efficacy. Whilst the need for ongoing randomized controlled trials examining the efficacy and safety of CAM undoubtedly exists, health services research is also important in order to gain an insight into the prevalence of CAM use, the profile and characteristics of CAM users, determinants of use and the interface between CAM and conventional medicine (Adams, 2007b). Beyond questions of prevalence and user characteristics there is a need to evaluate decision-making, information sources, access to CAM treatments and products, and treatment outcomes following CAM use.

This information will inform consumers, health care professionals, governments and health care policy makers (Adams, 2008). Health services research was listed as a new research goal in the US National Centre for

Complementary and Alternative Medicine's (NCCAM) 2005-2009 strategic plans (Herman, D'Huyvetter, & Mohler, 2006). A 2006 literature review of health 8 services research studies in CAM found 84 published studies (Herman, D'Huyvetter, & Mohler, 2006). Herman et al (2006) commented that many areas were, as yet, under explored and welcomed more research evaluating the many aspects of health services research in this area including the integration of CAM with orthodox medicine; development of patient guidelines; health insurance for CAM treatments; cost-effectiveness of CAM together with the adoption of whole systems research (the evaluation of a 'whole' system approach such as naturopathy, Ayurveda or traditional Chinese medicine) (Ritenbaugh, Verhoef, Fleishman, Boon, & Leis, 2003; Verhoef et al., 2005).

Prominent authors in the CAM field have called for more health services research to be conducted to examine the use of CAM in pregnancy, using large-scale, nationally representative samples of pregnant women in order to guide practice and policy development (Adams & Steel, 2012; Hall, Griffiths, & McKenna, 2011). Research is needed to quantify and characterize the profile of women who choose to use CAM products and visit CAM practitioners for pregnancy-related health issues. Pregnant women's attitudes towards the use of CAM during pregnancy as well as patterns of CAM use and influential sources of information in relation to this use are crucial to understanding and fully exploring the use of CAM during pregnancy (Adams & Steel, 2012; Steel & Adams, 2011; Hall et al., 2011).

This thesis provides one direct first step to responding to these important calls to address health services research gaps, using 9 well-recognized research methods and providing a novel contribution and advance to our understanding of CAM use during pregnancy.

11. CAM use in Taiwan

Traditional Chinese medicine has been the main medical treatment since the Ming and Ching Dynasties (AD 1368-1911) in both Taiwan and mainland China (Chi, 1994). Mental illness is traditionally regarded as a punishment for violating Confucian norms governing interpersonal relations, especially filial piety (Lin & Lin, 1981). Chinese culture believes in filial piety, a major aspect of Confucianism. Children learn to respect and obey their older family members. Violation of such values is believed to incur divine wrath that results in mental illness. As a result, when older people suffer from mental illness, the family unit may feel guilty and seek divine forgiveness by using folk religion, prayer or traditional healing in order to relieve or eradicate abnormal behaviors or mental illness (Ng, 1990). The family unit may also try many different kinds of treatment for the disease. Thus, Taiwanese people with health 3 problems often seek help from folk religion (Ng, 1990; Tsoi, 1985).

Religious or spiritual activities, such as traditional healing, may also be sought in Chinese culture for the treatment of mental illness. Chinese people may consult healers to use religious or traditional fool 4 Japanese policies on Chinese medicine were modified, allowing Chinese medicine to coexist with conventional medicine. In 1949 the Department of Health in Taiwan was established within the Ministry of the Interior to handle health care matters for the country (Committee on Chinese Medicine and Pharmacy Department of Health Taiwan, 2002). With the advancement of knowledge and globalization, Taiwan has been challenged to meet increasing demands from its population for better quality healthcare and lifestyle. The steady development of resources in healthcare is seen to be one of the most effective ways to improve the well-being of the Taiwanese people.

Indeed, the wide acceptance of CAM use by the public in Taiwan has been acknowledged as sufficiently overwhelming to challenge the government's policy on health care and contribute to the development of an integration of CAM with conventional medicine. The Taiwanese government stress flexibility in its health care system, and conventional medicine and traditional Chinese medicine not only coexist but also interact and mingle to form a pluralistic health care system in Taiwan (Committee on Chinese Medicine and Pharmacy Department of Health Taiwan, 2002). It was, and continues to be, the government's mission to integrate a variety of CAM therapies into conventional medical practice (Committee on Chinese Medicine and Pharmacy Department of Health Taiwan, 2002). Such integration aims to develop a new model of Chinese medicine, to modernize Chinese medicine, and combine Chinese medicine with advanced conventional medicine for the purpose of holistic health care in hospitals (Committee on Chinese Medicine and Pharmacy Department of Health Taiwan, 2002). Such service models enable hospitals to create greater convenience and provide improved quality of care to all patients. The Taiwanese government strongly believes that the integration of CAM and conventional medicine will bring better life and health to the community.

Today, treatments such as acupuncture and herbal remedies are covered by the National Health Insurance [NHI] program in Taiwan. Health care expenditure has increased dramatically in Taiwan since the implementation of NHI (Tsai & Kung, 2001). Per capita health expenditure in Taiwan has increased more than eight-fold from NT\$2,805 in 1980 to NT\$23,419 in 2000 (Chiang, 2002), which includes both 5 CAM covered by the NHI and conventional medicine. A payment policy has also been made for all contracted providers of various kinds of health services.

Since the implementation of the NHI program in 1995, health care consumers have had the opportunity to choose the health care services they wish to receive, and formal referral arrangements are not required. Furthermore, many hospitals in Taiwan are beginning to offer Chinese medicine services alongside conventional medicine. The number of doctors of Chinese medicine in Taiwan have increased (Statistics and Analysis Department of Health The Executive Yuan Taiwan R.O.C., 2002), although the number of doctors of Chinese medicine is small when compared to medical physicians. In 2001 there were 3,979 traditional Chinese medicine practitioners and 30,562 medical physicians in Taiwan (Statistics and Analysis Department of Health The Executive Yuan Taiwan R.O.C., 2002).

Thus, it is apparent that in a developing country like Taiwan, with a population of 22 million, CAM plays an indispensable role in the Taiwanese health care system. CAM has its own historical and cultural traditions and has had a profound influence on the values and way of life of the Chinese people, and on the development of Taiwan and China's health care system today. People in Taiwan consider using CAM for health problems, including mental disorders, because of a belief that it may treat their disease.

However, there is little scientific evidence for many CAM methods.

12. Influence of CAM on conventional medicine

It is anticipated that the relationship between non-conventional and conventional medicine will be closer in the future (Kolstad et al., 2004). An increase in CAM use raises concern about patients' adherence to prescribed medication or the improper use of both CAM and prescribed medication. People use CAM in a variety of ways. There is a general agreement about the combined use of both CAM and conventional medicine in Taiwan. Close to one third of outpatients in Taiwan have experience with taking Chinese medicine and conventional medicine at the same time (Lee, 2002). Lee et al. (2004) compared the illness and help-seeking behaviors of outpatients with major depressive disorders (n = 40), and non-depressive minor mental disorders (n = 41), in Taiwan.

They found that both groups used Western physicians, psychiatrists, traditional Chinese medicine, and folk therapy together for treating depression. Such 6 use is partly because Chinese patients and family follow the medical doctor's orders, and they hesitate to ask questions about their treatment or medications to avoid appearing disrespectful toward doctors (Purnell & Paulanka, 1998). Taiwanese patients traditionally respect and trust health care professionals, especially medical practitioners and nurses (Purnell & Paulanka, 1998; Tseng, Lin, & Yeh, 1995). Taiwanese people may also believe that recovery could be faster if they use more than one therapy. Therefore, people in Taiwan may receive and take both prescribed medication from a psychiatrist and herbal medicine from a Chinese medicine practitioner. However, combining both approaches may not work synergistically, and the potential compatibility or incompatibility between CAM and conventional medicine is not clear.

This combination of both health treatments may exacerbate the patient's condition, as well as increase possible toxic effects. It is important that health professionals are aware that people may use CAM in addition to, or instead of, conventional medicine. This is more likely when people believe that conventional medicine cannot cure their disorder, when conventional medicine is associated with serious side effects, or the health problems are not easily managed by conventional medicine, such as mental disorders. People with depression are more likely to terminate their conventional treatment because of adverse or intolerable side effects caused by drugs or age-related physiological changes (Nolan & O'Malley, 1988; Tsai, 2001). Concerns about side effects may encourage people to try CAM because they assume that CAM is helpful and free of side effects. Potential antidepressant-herb interactions have been reported in Taiwan. A serious adverse drug interaction between local Chinese medications with some psychotropic medications has also been reported in Taiwan (Yang et al., 1999). A male patient with bipolar I disorder lost consciousness for more than 24 hours because of severe complications after combining two common Taiwanese herbs: Centella asiatica and Oxalis corymbosa with lithium and psychotropics. Metabolic acidosis, acute respiratory failure, rhabdomyolysis and acute renal failure resulted.

Although, the patient was discharged after two months admission, chronic renal insufficiency, anaemia, mild psychomotor retardation, and mild generalized muscular atrophy still existed at the time of discharge. Stockley (1994) and Shader and Greenblat (1985; 1988) also reported that ginseng may potentiate the effect of Monoamine Oxidase 7 Inhibitors (MAOIs) and haloperidol (Micozzi, 2002). Despite the potential for serious complications, a person taking a combination of CAM and conventional medicine for treating mental disorders is common in Taiwan (Lee, et al., 2004; Yang et al., 1999).

These studies highlight that research is needed to provide a better understanding of the prevalence of CAM use and the influence of CAM use on conventional medicine. CAM and depression Very few studies have specifically focused on CAM use by patients with a psychiatrist-diagnosed depression, thus CAM use from the depressed patients' perspective has been under-explored. Depression results in an increasing use of CAM in this population, resulting in a higher need for nurses to understand CAM use. Against a background of an increasing number of people using CAM, and a lack of available evidence of CAM use for patients with depression, the need for this research study is apparent. Depression in older people.Most developed world countries have accepted the chronological age of 65 years as a definition of 'elderly' or older person (World Health Organization, 2000a).

People aged 65 years and over are at a high risk of developing mental disorders (World Health Organization, 2001) and depression (Regier et al., 1984). The population in Taiwan is ageing rapidly and thisis a major public concern in the 21st century (Wu & Chuang, 2001). In Taiwan in 2002, 13.3% of the population were aged 50 – 64 years and 9% were over 65 years of age in 2002, up from 8.81% in 2001 (Department of Household Registration Affairs Ministry of the Interior, 2004). In

2004, 14.5% of the population was aged 50 – 64 years and 9.5% were over 65 years of age (Department of Household Registration Affairs Ministry of the Interior, 2004). Therefore, as the population ages, depression of the aged will demand more attention from health professionals. Depression is a chronic condition affecting a wide range of persons with heterogeneous demographic characteristics.

Importantly, depression can progress to become a chronic condition that is disabling and difficult to treat successfully. Inadequate treatment is a major reason for the high risk of relapse of depression. Of the individuals who have had at least two episodes of major depression, 70% to 90% will have a third episode (Depression Guideline Panel, 1993). Depression is the leading cause of disability worldwide (National Institute of Mental Health, 2001) and is also associated with suicide. Seventy percent of all suicides are associated with depression (Stoudemire, Frank, Hedemark, Kamlet, & Blazer, 1986).

Older people are more likely than younger people to commit suicide, and older depressed patients are more likely than their non-depressed peers to suffer from other major illnesses. Suicide due to psychological problems was the twelfth leading cause of death for people 9 prescription or under-prescribing of antidepressant medication would provide less relief to patients than traditional Chinese herbal medicines. As Wen (1989) and Yang et al. (1999) remind us, Taiwanese people seek and prefer traditional treatment through Chinese medicine for mental and psychological problems. Conventional medicine is often referred to as mainstream medicine in Taiwan. Compared to CAM, conventional medicine has been tested following rigorous and scientific examinations to ensure safety and effectiveness. Su et al. (2002) suggests that an urgent challenge for mental health professionals is to consider factors affecting patients' use of antidepressant medication, as this remains unclear in Taiwan. It may be that people with depression, because of the influence of culture, use CAM rather than conventional medicine.

Wen (1998) reviewed the literature related to the relationship between illness behavior, help-seeking behavior, mental health and treatment in Taiwan, and concluded that folk medicine and culture have a powerful influence on illness behavior and mental health. CAM is an historical and cultural feature of health care in Taiwan, and has a profound influence over the treatment of mental disorders for the Taiwanese people. Beliefs about the effects of spiritual practices have a significant influence on medication compliance in patients with schizophrenia in

Taiwan (Lan, Lin, & Shiau, 2002). CAM covers a wide range of therapies, most of which are guided by and firmly embedded within cultural and belief systems in many developing countries (World Health Organization, 2002).

A study conducted in Taiwan (Lin, Lu, & Chan, 2003) investigated traumatic severity, post-traumatic responses and help-seeking behaviours after the Chi-Chi earthquake among 2,294 students and 1,096 parents in the affected area. This earthquake occurred in 1999 with 2,412 people killed and 11,305 injured. It is not surprising that the most common treatment they sought for psychological trauma was "startle curing", a folk treatment from folk healers. Folk medicine was found to be more reliable and effective in reducing acute psychological trauma than help from psychiatrists and professional consultants at the beginning of the post earthquake period. Folk medicine has a high curative value among people in Taiwan, however, the therapeutic effect of some forms of CAM is not clear (Lin, 1996). 10 Treatment and diagnosis of depression in Taiwanese people is a challenge for health professionals. When clients and/or their families cannot accept a diagnosis of depression they often turn to CAM practitioners, or even fortune-tellers, to seek comfort or to understand the origin of the disease according to folk religion or other traditional explanations for mental illness (Lin, 1985).

Patients and family in Taiwan may seek treatment for mental disorders in temples devoted to the Gods, or from the local mediator of folk religion (Lin, 1996; Wen, 1989). Rites of passage and medical beliefs in Taiwan are unique. In some cases, people with mental disorders see conventional medical doctors only because it is suggested or advised by Taoist or Buddhist healers. This may reflect a cultural influence on treatment for mental health and poor insight about the nature of depression and treatment for depression, and indicates a need to communicate the expectations of CAM that exist among persons with depression.

13. The influencing factors on adherence attitudes toward antidepressant medication

Attitudes toward CAM were found to be a predictor of adherence attitudes toward antidepressant medication. Patients who used CAM or were interested in such methods also expressed a high positive adherence attitude toward antidepressant medication. Three variables: attitudes toward antidepressants, patient education about CAM and patient education about antidepressant medication, were also associated with adherence toward antidepressant medication. Recommendations this study has contributed to the body of knowledge about depressed patients' interests in CAM. It has raised issues that might benefit from further discussion and debate, in particular the professional development needs of mental health nurses, and 182 appropriate nursing educations to facilitate a greater contribution to patient education.

Adequate nursing education about CAM will increase the knowledge ability of mental health nurses. The findings of this study, considered in relation to other studies and developments overseas, form the basis of the following recommendations. Nursing education Participants identified nurses' general knowledge and understanding about CAM as being limited. The findings suggest that serious consideration be given to the education of nursing students and registered nurses about CAM. Continuing nursing education should offer nurses training and education on CAM, both to improve nurses' knowledge of CAM and to enable them to impart this knowledge to patients and family, as well as to identify potential benefits and harms of CAM. Continuing education aims for the practical application of professional development, standards and advice relevant to clinical situations.

Adequate continuing education about CAM would enable nurses to respond knowledgeably to any questions or concerns patients may have about CAM and treatment options. It will enable nurses to not only keep communication channels open with patients, but to also possess adequate knowledge of the nature and potential risks, benefits and interactions with conventional medicine. Effective communication about CAM use should include six main priorities: 1. always ask patients about what else they may be using for their depression. 2. Consider patient preferences and values regarding CAM. 3. Promote communication between patients and health professionals on decision making regarding CAM use if patients require this assistance. 4. Provide patient education about what they should expect from both antidepressant medication and/or CAM for the treatment of depression. 5. Respond to patients' complaints related to conventional medicine such as antidepressant use and arrange follow-up. 6. Make recommendations to relevant health professionals to revise patients' care plans. Recommendations for undergraduate and postgraduate nursing curricula are also made. Educational content at the postgraduate level should address advanced CAM 183 information such as evidence-based data on safety, ideology and cultural and philosophical congruence.

Educational content at undergraduate level might include: 1. Basic information about CAM therapies, for example the roles of CAM in the treatment of various illnesses, and communication skills to talk with patients about CAM. 2. Health-related cultural beliefs about CAM use to foster culturally appropriate health care and to promote well-being. 3. Utilisation of well-organized websites about CAM in order to provide helpful web-based resources for self-learning. Nursing practice Depressed people have unique needs in relation to CAM use, such as the use of CAM for spiritual needs and the promotion of well-being, and it is important to support the health care needs of these people. The following nursing care plan about CAM use in the clinical settings is made based on the findings of this study.

Nurses should: 1. Utilize the Code of Ethics for Nurses in Taiwan (The National Union of Nurses' Associations ROC, 1994), in conjunction with the Practice Guidelines for the Treatment of Patients with Major Depressive Disorder (American Psychiatric Association, 2000), the Purpose and Mission of the TTCMNA (Taiwan Traditional Chinese Medicine Nurse Association, 2002), and Position on the Role of Nurses in the Practice of Complementary and Alternative Therapies (American Holistic Nurses' Association, 2003), and Policy on Complementary Therapies in Nursing Practice (Holistic Nurses Association of New South Wales, 1998) to make decisions about CAM use with patients and/or other health professionals. 2. Undertake regular assessment of patients' CAM use. 3. Undertake a background check on the CAM used by patients and seek out scientific information and research data available to critically evaluate the CAM in regards to safety and appropriateness, as well as the possible influences of demographic characteristics on CAM use. 184 4. Acknowledge the possible benefits and risks of some forms of CAM therapies for depression. 5. Discuss with psychiatrists and/or traditional Chinese medicine practitioners, if possible, about patients' use of CAM for depression in order to assist patients to avoid complications and/or adverse drug interactions. 6. Use communication skills to talk with patients and family in order to bring about a more satisfactory treatment outcome that is mutually acceptable in respect to both patient preferences and values and health professionals' knowledge and suggestions in relation to antidepressant medication and/or CAM.

7. Listen and evaluate the patient's opinions and ideas about their care, their attitudes toward CAM use and reasons why they are likely to seek CAM. 8. Utilize professional knowledge to manage and resolve conflicting priorities in relation to CAM and antidepressant medication within the nursing care plan. 9. Acknowledge and respect the patient's decision about CAM use, including use of CAM and/or antidepressant medication. 10. Educate patients of the importance of finding a licensed and credible CAM practitioner(s) if CAM is chosen. 11. Encourage patients to give feedback regarding decisions about nursing care plans.

14. The use of complementary and alternative medicine by cancer patients

The use of Complementary and Alternative Medicine (CAM) among cancer patients is widespread and appears to be increasing. However, it is not clear whether patients use CAM as an 'alternative' to standard oncology care or as an adjunct to the conventional treatment they receive. This study reviews the role of CAM therapies in the management of cancer, from the view of both patients and health professionals and it highlights issues relating to the efficacy of CAM used by cancer patients. Most patients use CAM to 'complement' the conventional therapies of radiotherapy, chemotherapy, hormone therapy and surgery. Health professionals in general have expressed positive views when CAM is used 'complementarily' and not as an 'Alternative'. Results so far published have shown that CAM can contribute to improving the quality of life of cancer patients and their general well-being.

There has been a steady increase in the use of complementary and alternative medicine among cancer patients for the past decades. Among the early studies to ascertain the level of CAM use among cancer patients, Downer et al, reported that 16% of cancer patients surveyed in two hospitals in London admitted to using CAM. This figure is similar to an earlier report in which CAM use was reported at 13% in the USA. However, a recent survey of 127 cancer patients in the UK reported that 29% of their sampled population was using some form of CAM. In a systematic review of surveys on the use of CAM among cancer patients in 13 countries, Ernst and Cassileth reported a range of 7% to 64% of CAM use among the adult cancer population and the average of 31.4% across all the studies.

Some of the commonly used CAM included visualization, herbs, dietary treatment, meditation, relaxation, homeopathy, hypnotherapy and other mega vitamins. The data collection method used in individual studies was either by interviewing the patients or sending out questionnaires or both. Nine out of the twenty-six surveys were conducted by means of interviewing the patients, fifteen were through questionnaire and two of them employed both methods. The prevalence rate among the nine surveys conducted through interview ranged between 7% and 37% with only one recording a rate of 54% of which spiritual healing was part of the treatment specified. The fifteen other surveys conducted by means of questionnaire reported a prevalence rate of between 16% and 64%. A survey in 14 European countries on the use of

CAM among patients with hematological cancers showed that 36% of cancer patients in Europe have used one or more forms of CAM modalities. Similarly, a rate of 40% was reported in the USA after a cross-sectional study of 1904 patients who have previously been diagnosed with cancer. A 2002 National Health Interview survey was used in this study. The most popular CAM therapies used were herbal medicine, deep breathing and meditation. An earlier study conducted in the United States produced a similar prevalence rate of 42%. A survey conducted in Canada reported a 43% prevalence rate of CAM use among cancer patients. In New Zealand, a rate of 49% among 200 cancer patients was reported. The most prominent of the therapies were Vitamins (68%) and Antioxidants (54%).

A similar result was found in Japan that found use among 44.6% of 3,100 cancer patients. However, 96.2% of the patients were using products such as Chinese herbs, mushroom, shark cartilage and vitamins, which would be considered as CAM products in the west. This emphasizes the problem with interpreting some of these data, as the reported varying prevalence rate of CAM use among cancer patients across different surveys has been attributed to the lack of consistency in the definition of CAM and its specificity with regard to what can be considered as a CAM modality. For example, Mao et al included prayer as a CAM modality, while others like Harris et al and Scott et al did not. Mao et al reported that over 61% of patients in his study relied on prayer as a form of CAM therapy for their cancer.

This is in contrast with a report which mentioned meditation and relaxation as the most commonly used CAM modality. However, the exclusion of prayer from the patients' questionnaire could be a factor. In a study in the UK, aromatherapy and relaxation techniques were among the most popular CAM therapies used by cancer patients. This is clearly in contrast to a survey where herbal medicines were reported to be the most commonly used therapy.

Despite these inconsistencies, the socio-demographic pattern of CAM use reveals some consistencies across most of the studies conducted on CAM use among cancer patients. The main recurring themes throughout most of the studies were that those who were most likely to use CAM were female, married people, higher earners, better educated and those who have used CAM before their diagnoses. In a study to assess the patterns of alternative medicine use by 319 cancer patients in Australia discovered that most of the patients who employed CAM as part of their cancer management were women (55.5%), people who were married (67.2%) and those with private health insurance (55.2%). This was consistent with the study carried out in Japan, which had women as the highest single users of CAM modalities in their study of 3100 cancer patients.

In the study by Downer et al, 52% of the sample populations who have admitted using a form of CAM were women, while 64% of the patients using complementary therapy were married. The study conducted by Molassiotis et al on CAM use among patients with hematological malignancies had 76% of the study sample as married, and over half of sample was women as well. These results may reflect the fact that breast cancer patients are the most likely group to use CAM therapies.

As more cancer patients turned to CAM in their quest to find a cure for their illness or to better their quality of life, the need to understand their views or perceptions of CAM is of interest. Ernst explained that the reasons given by patients for their use of CAM could be grouped into push factors (negative) which pushes patients away from conventional medicine and pull factors (positive) which relates to the positive aspects of CAM which makes it attractive to patients. Among the push factors are dissatisfaction with conventional medicine, the perceived "poor relationship" with some health care professionals, and desperation on the part of patients to get cured. Hope for a positive outcome of a treatment was mentioned as among some of the positive factors in addition to patients hope for a control over their treatment. Ernst also mentions that good rapport between patients and therapist, as well as the ease at which one can access a CAM modality is a determining factor for patients' use of CAM.

These reasons reflect those given by patients in various studies. Prominent among these were the urge to take control of the treatment and to improve their general condition. In a Norwegian study conducted to ascertain the reasons behind cancer patients' use of non-proven complementary therapies, 36% of 104 patients who participated reported actual improvement in their general condition.

The perceptions of patients regarding the use of CAM have been at the center of discussions whether it is used as an 'alternative' to standard oncology treatments of radiotherapy, surgery and chemotherapy or to 'complement' the conventional treatments. Regardless of whether patients use CAM as an 'Alternative' or 'Complementary' to conventional medicine, they perceive it as a very 'natural therapy' and 'harmless'. In a study by Penholder et al on the frequent use of complementary medicine by prostate cancer patients, 90% of the patients were reported to have used CAM with the aim to improve their quality of life. This view is supported by Roberts et al as well Kasha. In a Norwegian survey, it was reported that most patients were using CAM as it might give them strength to go through the conventional therapies and help to relieve their symptoms.

Molassiotis et al conducted a descriptive cross-sectional survey on 127 colorectal cancer patients across seven European countries. Over 47% of the patients reported using CAM with the view of increasing the body's ability to fight off the disease while just fewer than 45% of patients believed that CAM could help improve their physical well-being.

In a study by Begbie et al, the most common reason for CAM use was a new hope for cure (49%) and preference for 'natural therapy' was about 20%. Psychological distress was mentioned by Ernst and Fugh-Berma and Holland as among the popular reasons for patients using CAM. In a study on CAM use by cancer patients in Wales, patients cited pain relief as the main reason for using CAM.

Despite the fact that more and more cancer patients are turning to CAM modalities for a number of reasons, few patients disclose this to their health care professionals. Studies so far conducted by indicated that just about half of the cancer patients who use CAM inform their doctors of such use. Patients perceive a lack of interest on the part of health care professionals or their total disapproval of the therapies. The lack of communication about CAM between patients and health professionals limits the opportunity to discuss the potential benefits and risk of the therapies.

Complementary and Alternative Medicine (CAM) is defined by the Cochrane collaboration as:" a broad domain of healing resources that encompasses all health system, modalities, and practices and their accompanying theories and beliefs, other than intrinsic to the politically dominant health systems of a particular society or culture in a given historical period". However, the National Centre for Complementary and Alternative Medicine (NCCAM 2006) in America defines CAM as "a group of diverse medical and health care systems, practices and products that are not presently considered to be part of conventional medicine". The definition given by Cochrane emphasizes healing resources together with its beliefs and theories, while

NCCAM talks about systems, practices and products outside conventional medicine.

A more recent definition of CAM adapted by the Cochrane School of Complementary medicine is: " diagnosis, treatment and/or prevention which complements main stream medicine by contributing to a common whole, by satisfying a demand not met by orthodox methods or by diversifying the conceptual framework of medicine". Ernst and Cassileth favor this definition because it sees CAM as "complementary" to conventional medicine. The World Health Organization (WHO) defines CAM as: "A comprehensive term used to refer to both traditional medical systems such as traditional Chinese medicine, Indian Ayurveda, Arabic umami medicine, and to various forms of indigenous medicine".

The term Complementary and Alternative Medicine (CAM) is an umbrella term covering both 'complementary therapies' and 'alternative medicines'. Though the phrases are sometimes used synonymously, differences exist between the two. The phrase 'complementary therapy' is defined by cancerBacup as "treatments which are given alongside the conventional cancer treatments". This means it is there to complement the main conventional therapies such as radiotherapy, surgery, hormone treatment and chemotherapy in the case of cancer patients. The phrase 'Alternative medicine' is described as "practices used instead of standard medical treatment".

However, the definition of "Alternative medicine" outlined by World Health Organization (WHO) encompasses all forms of healthcare provision, which usually lie outside the official health sector. This definition makes no distinction between the terms "Alternative" and "Complementary". Therefore, in the case of cancer management, anything that falls outside radiotherapy, surgery, hormone therapy and chemotherapy could be considered as Alternative medicine. Because of the meaning attached to the phrase "Alternative therapy", most people prefer to use the term "complementary" instead, although the term is still used to differentiate natural medicine from modern medicine. Nonetheless, the term "Alternative medicine" is popular and much preferred in the United States, as most people still believe that it can sometimes replace conventional medicine in cases where conventional medicine has not lived to expectations.

Defining what complementary and alternative medicine (CAM) is, has not been without difficulties. One such problem lies in the fact that there is no clear-cut definition of CAM. What is considered as complementary in the UK is in fact conventional in another country. For instance, Lewith explains that herbal medicine and acupuncture are practiced as Complementary therapy in UK and USA whereas they are considered as part of the main conventional medicine in China.

According to CancerBacup, CAM can be divided into three different categories. These are psychological and self-help therapies, which help patients, deal with the emotional and psychological aspects of their illness like stress, anxiety and depression. Among these therapies are counseling, relaxation, healing, visualization, meditation and art therapy and hypnotherapy. The second groups of complementary therapies are considered as physical therapies. These therapies use the sense of touch as the main tool and among them are aromatherapy, acupuncture, massage, reflexology and shiatsu. The last group of complementary therapies is those classified as unconventional medicine or drugs, and includes Homeopathy, Herbal medicine, Essie, and Bach flower remedies.

However, Montbriand in his study on the overview of complementary therapies chosen by cancer patients had a different grouping for complementary therapies, and described the three types of CAM as psychological, physical and spiritual. The psychological therapies involve some kind of distraction strategies to take the mind of patients off the illness with a positive attitude towards life and finally cure. The physical therapies include herbal tea treatment, injection of thyme enzyme for the enhancement of the immune system, diet alteration and megavitamins. Spiritual therapies involve prayer and healing, for example.

It has been argued that Complementary and Alternative Medicine emphasizes the healing of both body and mind. According to Herzberg "While scientific medicine focuses on cures of diseases, complementary medicine is concerned with helping us to heal ourselves" Similarly Fulder, considers that complementary therapy emphasizes the restoration of health rather than the removal of sickness. Tschudin, points out that attitude is one of the fundamental differences between complementary therapies and orthodox medicine.

While orthodox or conventional medicine views symptoms as hostile and treats them accordingly, Tschudin considers that complementary therapies "use a symptom of illness which a person presents merely as a tool, guide or instructor, to discover more basic imbalances in the person's body, mind or spirit".

15. The history of alternative medicine

Heather acupuncture from China, Ayurveda therapies from India, or homeopathy in Europe, in her scholarly book, Roberta Bivins presents the belief systems that gave rise to such ancient practices and then follows their subsequent problematic global voyages to other cultures. Neither an allopathic doctor nor an alternative practitioner, Bivins provides readers with a social examination of these "exotic" techniques, from moxabustion to mesmerism, and explains how each was introduced (and then studied, simulated, ridiculed, or rejected) by Western physicians in Europe and the United States. The nearly four-century transcontinental propagation was not always easy — especially when corresponding belief systems could not be transported along with the therapeutic techniques.

The basis of many premodern medical practices rested on the belief that the human body was a microcosm of the universe. For instance, without the benefit of anatomical dissection (which was then amoral and illegal) or microscopic analysis (which was then unavailable), the acupuncturists in ancient China believed there were 12 waterways in the body that mirrored the country's 12 great rivers and canals. Ayurvedic medical practitioners believed in a deep philosophical and cosmological spiritual world of reincarnation and karma. A person's balanced and healthy interactions with the environment were necessary not only for the body but also for the soul. The translation of these principles and techniques from East to West paralleled the interaction of the cultures themselves, with all the inherent stereotyping, superstitions, and feelings of racial and cultural superiority. Ultimately, despite British imperialism or the medical profession's turf wars, it was often the realities of — and the lack of therapies for — epidemics of cholera and the plague, or ailments such as gout, that encouraged quick investigation and resulted in rejection or eventual co-optation of the unfamiliar treatments. Of note, the authorities investigating and discounting alternative therapies were also often "borrowing" the practices for reintroduction as their own. One example was moxabustion, a therapy that uses heat and was apparently effective in the treatment of gout.

During the 18th and 19th centuries, the Western medical establishment was looking with a critical eye at the use of Chinese herbs and the practice of homeopathy while practicing what it knew as the best standards of care — cupping and bleeding. Some ancient practices were later "discovered" in the West. Centuries before Edward Jenner determined that mild cowpox exposure conferred immunity to smallpox, Asians practiced variolation — the controlled exposure to a carefully selected mild case of smallpox in one person to produce immunity in another. This same practice is followed today by some parents, who bring their unimmunized children to chicken pox or measles parties.

Early remedies paved the way for later advances. Acupuncture was not readily adopted by Western doctors, but Bivins speculates that acupuncture helped to familiarize them with needles, domesticating needles for later use in vaccines, drug delivery, and the drawing of blood. There are important lessons in this book for practicing physicians. For example, techniques such as homeopathy may have become popular not because of consistent efficacy but because the patients appreciated attentive clinicians and were attracted to the treatment's benign nature and affordability.

The Western physician, past and present, is made out to be mostly predatory and misguided. Bivins questions why researchers continue to assess treatments from other cultures in a Western framework. Admittedly, we do not have the technology to measure qi or to visualize prana (which of course does not disprove their existence), but we do have the tools to objectively evaluate clinical interventions. With 60% of U.S. medical schools now offering some instruction in alternative medicine, and the commitment to research being made by the National Institutes of Health's National Center for Complementary and Alternative Medicine, there is an effort under way to evaluate practices that may hold promise and bring them into our evidence-based world.

Bivins's book is a work of scholarship filled with thoughtful discussion, but it is largely devoid of colorful or memorable characters, a clear timeline or plot, or clinical discussions — all of which would have made the book more appealing. Bivins does ask one provocative question, illustrated in part by the use of a question mark in the book's title: Why do we continue to use the word "alternative" when the popularity and complementary integration of some of these therapies, especially for the treatment of chronic conditions, continues to increase? There are now more patient visits to alternative medical practitioners than to primary care physicians in the United States.

In the end, this book is about Western attitudes toward the non-Western world. It is a macroscopic analysis rich with philosophical reflection and historical observation that exposes the difficulty of exporting such therapies outside their original cultures and belief structures.

One of the oldest forms of alternative medicine can be traced back through Chinese history. The ancient Chinese, in much the same way as alternative medicine, is used today, based their healing on the importance of the body and spirit being in balance. Much of the philosophy of Chinese Medicine is based on Taoist and Buddhist principals and the belief that a person and their environment are closely interlinked. The widely known principles of Yin and Yang come from Chinese Medicine and are integral to its practice.

Yin and Yang explain how opposing forces are integral to each other and how for harmony within the body to take place, these must be in balance. When these are out of balance, disease occurs. Chinese Medicine works at restoring balance in various ways including herbal medicine, acupuncture, breathing and movement (Tai Chi and Qigong) and also through diet. The practitioner looked at the patient's health and life in detail to ascertain where their life force or Qi (pronounced Chi) was out of balance. Various methods would then be used to restore the patient back to health. Such was the effectiveness of Chinese Traditional Medicine that it still forms a large part of modern health care in the East. It's not unusual for these alternative practices to be used in hospitals alongside western medicine.

The result now is that Alternative Medicine is on the increase. Practices such as acupuncture, herbal medicine, aromatherapy, and healing are kept alive by practitioners who specialize in one or more alternative form of treatment. Frequently alternatives are used alongside modern medical treatments, which have led to alternatives being given the term complementary medicine. These brief histories of alternative medicine shows that many of the practices used today have been with us for thousands of years. Given the rising popularity of using alternative medicine to deal with health issues today, it's likely that these practices will be around for many more.

The history of alternative medicine refers to the history of a group of diverse medical practices that were collectively promoted as "alternative medicine" beginning in the 1970s, to the collection of individual histories of members of that group, or to the history of western medical practices that were labeled "irregular practices" by the western medical establishment. It includes the histories of complementary medicine and of integrative medicine. "Alternative medicine" is a loosely defined and very diverse set of products, practices, and theories that are perceived by its users to have the healing effects of medicine, but do not originate from evidence gathered using the scientific method, are not part of biomedicine, or are contradicted by scientific evidence or established science. "Biomedicine" is that part of medical science that applies principles of anatomy, physics, chemistry, biology, physiology, and other natural sciences to clinical practice, using scientific methods to establish the effectiveness of that practice.

Much of what is now categorized as alternative medicine was developed as independent, complete medical systems, was developed long before biomedicine and use of scientific methods, and was developed in relatively isolated regions of the world where there was little or no medical contact with pre-scientific western medicine, or with each other's systems. Examples are Traditional Chinese medicine, European humeral theory and the Ayurvedic medicine of India. Other alternative medicine practices, such as homeopathy, were developed in Western Europe and in opposition to western medicine, at a time when western medicine was based on unscientific theories that were dogmatically imposed by western religious authorities. Homeopathy was developed prior to discovery of the basic principles of chemistry, which proved homeopathic remedies contained nothing but water.

But homeopathy, with its remedies made of water, was harmless compared to the unscientific and dangerous orthodox western medicine practiced at that time, which included use of toxins and draining of blood, often resulting in permanent disfigurement or death. Other alternative practices such as chiropractic and osteopathic manipulative medicine, were developed in the United States at a time that western medicine was beginning to incorporate scientific methods and theories, but the biomedical model was not yet totally dominant. Practices such as chiropractic and osteopathic, each considered to be irregular by the medical establishment, also opposed each other, both rhetorically and politically with licensing legislation. Osteopathic practitioners added the courses and training of biomedicine to their licensing and licensed Doctor of Osteopathic Medicine holders began diminishing use of the unscientific origins of the field, and without the original practices and theories, is now considered the same as biomedicine.

Until the 1970s, western practitioners that were not part of the medical establishment were referred to "irregular practitioners", and were dismissed by the medical establishment as unscientific or quackery. Irregular practice became increasingly marginalized as quackery and fraud, as western medicine increasingly incorporated scientific methods and discoveries, and had a corresponding increase in success of its treatments. In the 1970s, irregular practices were grouped with traditional practices of nonwestern cultures and with other unproven or disproven practices that were not part of biomedicine, with the group promoted as being "alternative medicine".

Following the counterculture movement of the 1960s, misleading marketing campaigns promoting "alternative medicine" as being an effective "alternative" to biomedicine, and with changing social attitudes about not using chemicals, challenging the establishment and authority of any kind, sensitivity to giving equal measure to values and beliefs of other cultures and their practices through cultural relativism, adding postmodernism and DE constructivism to ways of thinking about science and its deficiencies, and with growing frustration and desperation by patients about limitations and side effects of science-based medicine, use of alternative medicine in the west began to rise, then had explosive growth beginning in the 1990s, when senior level political figures began promoting alternative medicine, and began diverting government medical research funds into research of alternative, complementary, and integrative medicine.

Conclusion

Complementary and Alternative Medicine is an increasingly popular option among cancer patients. However, lack of clear definitions about what constitutes CAM makes it difficult to reach clear conclusions about efficacy and safety. Even so, there is no evidence to suggest that CAM can replace conventional treatment, and there is a need for reliable and consistent information to be made available to patients.

CAM is becoming more significant among the increasing numbers of people and clients using it. Where patients have had access to CAM, it is anticipated that they will seek alternatives or complementary therapies to enhance what they consider as more than optimal care. CAM within the healthcare system is an important component and requires careful consideration since it plays a key role in a person's overall health and will increasingly assume a more significant place in the overall management of nursing practice. 176 This study sought to explore CAM use among patients with depression in Taiwan and the impact that demographic, attitudinal and educational factors exerted on CAM use. The study also sought to identify those factors that influenced decision-making and behaviour in relation to adherence to antidepressant medication. The significance of the study is therefore in the contribution it makes to the current level of knowledge in relation to CAM use by patients with depression in Taiwan. Patients seek and make their own judgments about what constitutes holistic and patient-centered health care. Most patients are willing to accept CAM as part of their depression management. Thus, the outcomes for patients and nurses are significant.

It is important that the nursing profession has a clear understanding of patients' use of CAM. Opportunities need to be provided for patients with depression to talk throughout the entire treatment period, gain a better understanding of their decision making about their plan, and express their feelings and concerns in relation to depression treatment, both conventional and alternative or complementary. The findings indicate that CAM use is affected by multiple factors. These factors may be considered by the nursing profession in future educational and research planning. The study findings suggest a number of implications, described in the next chapter, as recommendations for quality use of CAM, practice, education, and further research.

CAM is to educate patients about the uncertainties of CAM use with and without antidepressant medication, what they should expect to happen when they begin the treatment, and possible herb-drug interactions. For example, whether CAM use will conflict with antidepressant treatment, or whether CAM can cure depression. Patients need to understand that while CAM may well have a role to play; it is not a treatment for depression in its own right. There is emerging evidence as detailed in Chapters 2 and 6 that CAM therapies such as relaxation techniques, massage and yoga are likely to have some benefits for depressive mood. Furthermore, spiritual healing may also offer depressed patients emotional support. Patients should be informed of the following principles of CAM use to assist their decision-making: It is important to tell patients to consider conventional medicine options first as antidepressant medications have been shown to be effective in treatment of depression (American Psychiatric Association, 2000).

If CAM is accepted as a part of patients' health care plans, then they need to communicate this information to their treating health professional. CAM may be useful for low intensity symptoms in the absence of other, more effective treatments, and when the specific CAM therapy has been scientifically proven to be safe and effective.

Alternative medicine is the term for medical products and practices that are not part of standard care. Standard care is what medical doctors, doctors of osteopathy, and allied health professionals, such as nurses and physical therapists, practice. Alternative medicine is used in place of standard medical care. An example is treating heart disease with chelation therapy (which seeks to remove excess metals from the blood) instead of using a standard approach. Examples of alternative practices include homeopathy, traditional medicine, chiropractic, and acupuncture. Complementary medicine is different from alternative medicine. Whereas complementary medicine is used together with conventional medicine, alternative medicine is used in place of conventional medicine. See also complementary medicine, conventional medicine.

Something big is happening in healthcare, and it's centered on a desire to have different options within healthcare that considers the whole person. This demand is being filled by alternative medicine and a growing base of practitioners who are dedicated to leading the holistic healthcare movement. For instance, in 2012, Americans spent over $30 billion on alternative medicine. An estimated 59 million Americans spent an average of $500 per person on complementary and alternative medicine (CAM).

From yoga to nutritional supplements to acupuncture, consumers across the nation are seeking alternatives to pharmaceutical drugs and surgery. As studies continue to emerge that point to the validity of these alternative treatments, the CAM movement is gaining momentum without a slowdown in sight.

References

-WHO, Fact sheet N°134, 2008, http://www.who.int/mediacentre/factsheets/2003/fs134/en/.

-A. Gurib-Fakim, "Medicinal plants: traditions of yesterday and drugs of tomorrow," Molecular Aspects of Medicine, vol. 27, no. 1, pp. 1–93, 2006. View at Publisher · View at Google Scholar · View at Scopus

-V. Chintamunnee and M. F. Mahomoodally, "Herbal medicine commonly used against infectious diseases in the tropical island of Mauritius," Journal of Herbal Medicine, vol. 2, pp. 113–125, 2012. View at Google Scholar

-H. Nunkoo and M. F. Mahomoodally, "Ethno pharmacological survey of native remedies commonly used against infectious diseases in the tropical island of Mauritius," Journal of Ethnopharmacology, vol. 143, no. 2, pp. 548–564, 2012.

-Amira OC, Okubadejo NU. 'Frequency of Complementary and Alternative Medicine Utilization in Hypertensive Patients Attending an Urban Tertiary Care Centre in Nigeria' BMC Complementary and Alternative Medicine. 2007;7(30):1–5.

-Amzat J, Abdullahi A A. 'Role of Traditional Healers in the Fight against HIV/AIDS' EthnoMed. 2008;2(2):153–159.

- Bamidele J O, Adebimpe W O, Oladele E A. 'Knowledge, Attitude and Use of Alternative Medical Therapy amongst Urban Residents of Osun State, Southwestern Nigeria' African Journal of Traditional and Complementary/ Alternative Medicine. 2009;6(3):281–288.

-Banjo A D, Lawal O A, Owolana O A, Ashidi J S, Dedeke G A, Soewu D A, Owara S O, Sobowale O A. 'An Ethnozoological Survey Of Insects And Their Allies Among The Remos (Ogun State) South Western Nigeria' Indilinga African Journal of Indigenous Knowledge System. 2003;2:61–68.

-Bello R A. 'Integrating the Traditional and Modern Health Care System in Nigeria: A Policy Option for Better Access to Health Care Delivery' In: Saliu H, Jimoh A, Arosanyin T, editors. The National Question and Some Selected Topical Issues on Nigeria. Ibadan: Vantage Publishers; 2006.

- Blench R, Dendo M. 'Fulfulde names for plants and trees in Nigeria Cameroun, Chad and Niger', Cambridge. 2006a. (accessed from http://www.rogerblench.info/Ethnosciencedata/FulfuldePlantnames.pdf on the 8th September, 2009)

-Cameron A, Ewen M, Ross-Degnan D, Ball D, Laing R. Medicine Prices, Availability, and Affordability in 36 Developing and Middle-Income Countries: A Secondary Analysis. Geneva: The World Health; 2008.

- Carpentier L, Prazuck T, Vincent-Ballereau F, Ouedraogo L T, Lafaix C. 'Choice of Traditional of Modern Treatment in West Burkina Faso. World Health Forum. 1995;16:198–210.

-Chatora R. 'An Overview of the Traditional Medicine Situation in the African Region' African Health Monitor. 2003;4(1):4–7. [

-Ajzen, I., & Fishbein, M. (1980). Understanding attitudes and predicting social behaviour. Englewood Cliffs: Prentice-Hall. Akdemir, A., Turkcapar, M. H., Orsel, S. D., Demirergi, N., Dag, I., & Ozbay, M. H. (2001).

- Reliability and validity of the Turkish version of the Hamilton Depression Rating Scale. Comprehensive Psychiatry, 42(2), 161-165.

-Alberta Association of Registered Nurses. (1999). Standards for registered nurses: Alternative and complementary therapy in nursing practice. Retrieved April 27, 2005, from http://www.nurses.ab.ca/pdf/Standards

-Ajzen, I., & Fishbein, M. (1980). Understanding attitudes and predicting social behaviour. Englewood Cliffs:

Prentice-Hall. Akdemir, A., Turkcapar, M. H., Orsel, S. D.,
Demirergi, N., Dag, I., & Ozbay, M. H. (2001).
-Reliability and validity of the Turkish version of the
Hamilton Depression Rating Scale. Comprehensive
Psychiatry, 42(2), 161-165.

-Alberta Association of Registered Nurses. (1999).
Standards for registered nurses: Alternative and
complementary therapy in nursing practice. Retrieved April
27, 2005, from http://www.nurses.ab.ca/pdf/Standards_

.

www.ingramcontent.com/pod-product-compliance
Lightning Source LLC
Chambersburg PA
CBHW030624220526
45463CB00004B/1409